MIDLIFE TUNE-UP

MIDLIFE TUNE-UP

SIX SIMPLE STEPS

TIM BURNS

PELICAN PUBLISHING COMPANY
GRETNA 2006

*The word "Pelican" and the depiction of a pelican
are trademarks of Pelican Publishing Company, Inc.,
and are registered in the U.S. Patent and Trademark Office.*

Library of Congress Cataloging-in-Publication Data

Burns, Tim.
  Midlife tune-up : six simple steps / Tim Burns.
    p. cm.
  ISBN-13: 978-1-58980-396-1 (hardcover : alk. paper)
  1. Middle-aged persons—Religious life. 2. Middle-aged
persons—Employment. 3. Success—Religious aspects—
Christianity.
  I. Title.
  BV4579.5.B88 2006
  155.6'6—dc22
                                                    2006019008

Printed in the United States of America
Published by Pelican Publishing Company, Inc.
1000 Burmaster Street, Gretna, Louisiana 70053

To Karen, the spark in my life

Contents

MIDLIFE TUNE-UP

PART 1

Confronting Midlife

CHAPTER 1

The Midlife Wakeup Call

Adversity is the first path to truth.
   —Lord George Noel Gordon Byron, Don Juan

Life begins at forty.

         —Anonymous

The mass of men lead lives of quiet desperation.
      —Henry David Thoreau, Walden

My Call

The pang of midlife can strike when you least expect it, piercing you with a jolt of sadness, remorse, and yearning. For me it occurred quite unexpectedly on the last day of the entrepreneurship class that I was teaching at the A. B. Freeman School of Business at Tulane University, while the undergraduate students were presenting their business-plan projects.

As each of the fresh-faced students effortlessly downloaded their PowerPoint files from their Internet mailboxes for presentation on the built-in LCD projector, the blackboard, which had been the staple in my learning process, seemed pathetically awkward and ignored as it relinquished center stage to the retractable screen in this digital age of learning.

One of the business plans concerned an entertainment service that targeted "young" patrons, those between the ages of twenty and thirty-five, for trendy bars and restaurants in New Orleans. I was a decade beyond the target group. Although I struggled to pay attention to the fine points of their presentations, my mind strayed. I had always enjoyed teaching and had taught for years, mostly to adults who were older than myself. But returning to my alma mater to teach undergraduates for the first time had a profound impact on me. Although there were many new buildings on campus, including the impressive new structure that now housed the business school, Tulane still had the same "feel" that I remembered from many years earlier.

I had graduated prior to cell phones, pagers, laptop computers, palm pilots, and even fax machines. The only computer I ever used was the centralized mainframe that ran the entire university and required typed cards to harness its processing power, then probably a fraction of a single laptop sitting in a student's dormitory room today.

What had happened? Over two decades had dribbled away. It seemed only yesterday I was scuttling around Tulane's treelined campus with my knapsack, slipping sheepishly into one of the wooden desks in the back of the traditional classroom, often after class had started, with my whole life and career ahead of me. Today, I was facing my own students, assuredly settled into comfortable swivel chairs in a tiered amphitheater that reminded me more of a corporate conference center than a college classroom. I often felt that my students were judging me as opposed to my grading them.

The presentations continued. One displayed the financial forecast for the business, which included a balance sheet. I thought about my own balance sheet. I had no spouse or serious romantic interest, my career was helplessly stalled, and my net worth had been decimated by the dot-com bust. I was once a young Tulane undergraduate, as cocky as many of the young men who sat in the back of the room and periodically made flip comments. But I was feeling anything but cocky lately . . . I felt downright helpless and miserable instead.

I finally realized that I wasn't being fair to my students. They had prepared for today and I needed to reward them with my complete attention. With a great heave, I pushed my depressing thoughts to the side and focused on their presentations.

At the end of class, several students lingered to wish me well and, of course, furtively mention that they enjoyed my class. A few of their comments seemed sincere. A piece of their college transcript and a small part of their lives rested in my hands. Yet it seemed that they had all the power, with their young lives ahead of them.

After the last student left, I sat in one of the swivel chairs and reflected. I remembered myself as an idealistic young student, thinking that the sky was the limit and planning to set the whole world on fire. Instead, I feared that I had crashed and burned, my present life only charred remains of what could have been.

I had done both my undergraduate and graduate work at Tulane and after eight hectic years had collected three degrees, including the trendy M.B.A./J.D.. Along the way I passed the CPA exam to add some icing to my résumé. I thought I was set for life.

For a while, it appeared that I might be right. Upon graduation, I slid almost effortlessly into an old-line, prestigious corporate law firm in New Orleans and was paid a top salary. Then, I parlayed my three years at the law firm into an even higher paying job with a Fortune 500 company that had recently relocated from New York to New Orleans and was looking to beef up its corporate law department. I charged into my new position with boundless enthusiasm. Soon, I was firmly entrenched in the corporate fast track, jetting around the world closing creative and complex deals that dwarfed anything that my contemporaries were doing and that required every ounce of my education, intelligence, and stamina. I was barely thirty years old but had already caught the attention of senior management. One particular transaction had added tens of millions of dollars to the company's bottom line and I had received much of the credit. But I was too busy to notice that I was working too much, neglecting my personal life and squeezing relationships in around my hectic work schedule. The only thing I cared about was that my career was going *great*, or so I thought.

Then came the transfer.

As the 1980s ended and the 1990s began, the company, like the rest of corporate America, initiated a process that was delicately called "restructuring." For a while, the layoffs and transfers were restricted to fringe areas, but then veered towards the heart of the company. Although I considered myself one of the more productive lawyers, I was sent packing from the legal department at the corporate headquarters in New Orleans to go to an unfilled governmental relations position at the State Capitol in Baton Rouge, primarily to prevent any reduction in the staffing of the legal department. Although I should have been grateful for surviving a particularly onerous "restructuring," I was not. As far as I was concerned, I had been unfairly plucked from my beloved and challenging arena of international deal making and exiled to a corporate outpost for a lobbying job for which I was overqualified, in a city in which I did not wish to live, and for a supervisor for whom I did not wish to work. I made other job inquiries but could not find as comfortable a place to land in a tight economy. I settled into my new job and did the best I could. The good news was that the interruption of my jet-setting pace and workaholism gave me the time to examine many issues in my life that had been sorely neglected and pursue other interests besides work. The layoffs continued at corporate headquarters, but I barely noticed them from my seemingly secure corporate outpost.

Then came the earthquake.

The company suddenly announced that, due to poor profits, it was shedding one-third of its workforce as well as most of its domestic assets, including those I had been hired to protect at the State Capitol. My complacency vanished as this new set of layoffs became as ominous as a swinging pendulum blade moving closer and closer to my formerly secure corporate outpost. I clung to the job I previously detested as if it were a life raft while I desperately searched for another position.

To my dismay, my experience, my accomplishments, and my education were generally ignored by corporate America. Much of my difficulty stemmed from the fact that other companies were also shedding employees at the time. The legal field in particular is notoriously difficult to laterally transfer within. The large law firms, for which I was best suited, tend to prefer fresh young minds that they can mold to their own liking. Such firms are only interested in adding experienced lawyers who bring along new business with them. I had not really practiced law for a number of years and had no clients of my own. But even though I was going against the grain, I came agonizingly close to several promising positions. One was with the branch office of a major law firm and the other as the head of a distinguished non-profit entity that served as a watchdog for state government.

In each case, I seemed assured of the position, only to have some last-minute complication botch the deal.

The branch office of the law firm was anxious to hire me and had in fact extended me an informal offer. But just as things were about to become formalized, a résumé showed up at the main office that the powers there felt was a better fit. The main office overruled the branch office and my offer vanished.

The nonprofit entity was even more of a heartbreak. Mine had started off as 1 of over 120 résumés submitted for the position of executive director of the high-profile entity, which advocated good government in Louisiana, a state that certainly experienced its share of bad government. The position was considered very prestigious, with its former executive director being tapped by a new governor as the commissioner of administration for the state of Louisiana, responsible for the entire operations of the state. I survived three cuts to eventually become one of five finalists. The position would have utilized my governmental relations experience and my business background as well as my legal expertise. I was excited by the challenge of taking this somewhat dormant but well-respected entity to new heights. I had prepared a lengthy position paper, and my interview with the search committee had gone extremely well. I had done my homework, and the committee members were outwardly impressed with my vision for the entity as well as my qualifications for the position. Although I was the youngest of the contenders, I had received word from insiders that my interview and résumé had made the best impression. The committee was scheduled to reconvene that day and would likely recommend me to the board.

However, that night, the retired, but still much respected, former chairman of the entity personally intervened on behalf of another finalist, who happened to be his protégé. Although some of the committee members purportedly had their doubts about the choice, the former chairman was apparently quite persuasive in calling in his chits. I found the promising job snatched from my hands at the last second. The protégé ended up lasting barely a year in the position.

Sixty days later I was laid off from my company. The good news was that I had a relatively soft landing. I was given a consulting contract with the company and ended up as "of counsel" with the law firm of a high-school classmate. The bad news was that I was forty and had to start all over again. I had no clients, had not practiced law for a number of years, and felt a bit out of place at the firm. My classmate and his partner, who were around my age, owned the firm, and the remaining associates were generally younger and more recent law graduates. My classmate was most gracious about the arrangement and often referred to me as the "smart kid" from the class. But if I was so "smart," how did I end up back at the starting gate with lawyers over a decade younger than me?

My career at the firm hobbled along. New clients were not easy to come by and I felt that I was barely holding my own and even losing some ground. I watched many clients get rich while I struggled to collect my hourly fees. I was making a living and that was about it.

My personal life also had its up and downs. In the years after graduation, I found myself in and out of unhealthy relationships that were the easiest to juggle around my career. But just about the time of my transfer by the company, I met a nice woman who had been recently divorced and I entered into my first serious relationship. Although my body was transferred to Baton Rouge, my heart remained in Mandeville (a New Orleans suburb north of Lake Pontchartrain, where she lived) and I became well acquainted with the stretch of highway that divided the two.

Other good things had happened. I started writing again, something I had not done since my college days. My new position with the company afforded travel opportunities in which guests were allowed to tag along. We traveled extensively both on and off the corporate expense account and generally had a good life together, particularly in the years after the transfer but before the earthquake. For a while I was actually fairly happy.

However, something that I did not completely understand prevented me from making that final commitment to her. We had sessions with a relationship counselor and even attended some couples' workshops. I prayed, meditated, and read everything I could on relationships. I even bought her an expensive engagement ring and checked into foreign wedding destinations. I did everything but set a wedding date. And as the weeks turned to months and the months turned to years, the love began to seep slowly away. She eventually moved away to pursue her long-cherished dream of living by the beach, even though she had emotionally departed the relationship years earlier.

My finances had not fared much better. Like everyone else, I had become enamored with the stock-market boom of the late 1990s, in particular the technology stocks. As the market began its downturn, I kept listening to my broker, who assured me that this was a temporary correction and everything would be okay. We all know now that the market slide for many technology high flyers was anything but a temporary correction.

I was more angry at myself than at my broker. Even though I had an M.B.A., I had allowed my personal and retirement portfolios to become dramatically undiversified and had ignored the same advice about risk allocation that any of my students could have told me from their first-year finance course. In other words, don't put all of your eggs in one basket. My net worth had been nearly decimated.

Maybe that was why I was feeling broke, alone, and unsuccessful these days. During this time, I had also lost three close family members: my grandmother, at the end of a very long and fruitful life; my father, after a battle with lung cancer; and my nephew, so tragically at the beginning of his young life that I can't really discuss it but only pray for my sister and her family.

My awareness returned to the empty classroom. Possibly the thought of real tragedy had extracted me from my self-pity. I was definitely in the throes of some midlife crisis, but whining about it was not going to do me any good. I felt utterly defeated.

My self-esteem had ebbed so low that I felt dependent on the "kindness of strangers." This phrase comes from the classic play *Streetcar Named Desire*, by Tennessee Williams, which is set in the New Orleans French Quarter. The words are spoken in a very dramatic scene by the pathetic and forlorn Blanche Dubois, who has been finally pushed over the edge after being raped by her beastly brother-in-law, Stanley Kowalski. In the movie version, Kowalski was played brilliantly by Marlon Brando (who can forget "Stell-ahhh!"?). When Blanche is finally being carted away to the asylum, it initially appears that she will have to be physically subdued. Then, the kindly doctor speaks reassuringly to her and offers her his arm. With his support, she makes her way out, saying, "Whoever you are, I have always depended on the kindness of strangers."

These days, I wasn't feeling in much better shape than poor Blanche. I felt I was drifting through life with no rudder or purpose. I would wake up thinking about things that didn't matter, talking to people who weren't there, and hoping that life would spare me for yet another day. I only felt good when someone said something nice, and such words of assurance were becoming increasingly harder to come by. My constant grumbling had drained my friends of any empathy, actually leaving me dependent on the kindness of strangers. Any negative comment or unkind action could send me into a tailspin. Criticism continued to pile up. I was constantly making mistakes, missing deadlines, offering excuses, and spinning myself silly in an ominous whirlpool that was sucking me under.

I had recently bumped into an old friend, who informed me that he was raising children, making money, and having fun. I responded that I was doing *none* of the above. I felt an utter lack of enthusiasm for life. I was simply going through the motions, often running from life rather than embracing it. I was scrambling to avoid failure as opposed to confidently pursuing success.

There were tears in my eyes. I placed my head down on the classroom table and hoped that nobody would walk in. How had my life turned out so badly? I had played by the rules. I studied hard and worked hard and generally did what I was supposed to do. What was the problem? How was I possibly going to get out of this? I didn't have a clue.

Then I remembered someone I had known a long time ago.

With his shaggy hair, blue jeans, and T-shirts, he wasn't that much to look at. He was actually a bit brash for my taste. He talked openly of his bold plans to obtain several degrees from an expensive private university when neither he nor his parents had any money. This whole idea seemed quite ludicrous under the circumstances. But the strange thing was that he succeeded. It wasn't easy and there were many setbacks along the way. But he persisted and somehow managed to complete his education. It had taken working three jobs at a time, student loans, and today's equivalent of $250,000 in scholarship assistance. But the truth is that he succeeded because he never once doubted that he would.

So I thought . . . if I did it then, I can do it now.

I felt a surge of positive energy and hope, deeper than I had experienced in a long time. I *had* succeeded in the past. I had beaten tremendous odds to complete my education. All of my friends in college had come from very wealthy households. My best friend's father owned one of the largest electronics manufacturers in the world. His family owned homes in New York City, Hong Kong, and Fort Lauderdale. When we would go through the school registration line together, he would pull out a blank check from his dad to pay the thousands of dollars in tuition, boarding, and fees. Most of my expenses were covered by scholarships and work study and I would fish the necessary cash out of my pocket to pay my bill of only a few hundred dollars. I was waiting tables back then and was paid in cash. Yet despite our different backgrounds and bank accounts, I was his classmate and his peer. Suddenly it became quite obvious to me what had been the key to my success in school.

Act As If You Cannot Fail

I retrieved a legal pad from my briefcase and wrote down: *Act as if you cannot fail.*

These days, I was acting as if failure was just around the corner. I had succeeded at Tulane because failure was simply not an option. I had never once doubted that I would succeed. My parents had struggled to send me to an expensive and elite grammar and high school. Many of my friends were going to Tulane and so was I. There was simply no way that I wasn't. I was totally confident in my quest for college and it showed.

Of course, there were many setbacks along the way. I was a Truman Scholarship finalist for the state of Louisiana but lost out on the prestigious and lucrative award. Another potential scholarship slipped through my fingers. I sometimes felt like giving up, but there was a stronger force inside me that refused to quit. I was quite relentless in my desire to finish school. When the front doors seemed closed, I tried the side doors. When the side doors were closed, I tried the back doors. I would've broken in if I would have had to. Eventually, I caught the breaks I needed. I found the scholarships and the jobs when I was low on funds. I took out student loans to cover other expenses. I was able to complete my undergraduate and graduate work on schedule, as I had planned years earlier. But the main reason I succeeded was because I acted as if I could not fail. Had I tried to scale that daunting educational summit any less confidently, I probably would have slipped down along the way.

As I sat in the campus classroom that night, I realized the ultimate irony of my success in completing my education. The confidence and perseverance behind my diplomas should have been the launching point for my career. Instead, they had been my high point. After graduation, I seemed to never approach obstacles and adversity nearly as resourcefully as I had during my student days. It was almost as if I had left much of my self-confidence behind at Tulane. Once I entered the workforce, fear and self-defeating behaviors crept into my life. Lately, I had allowed career difficulties and the ending of a long-term relationship to shatter my self-esteem and derail my life. I felt reduced to relying on chance and even the kindness of strangers to somehow put me back on track. Perhaps the skies would part and fortune would once again smile down upon me. I was looking for answers everywhere except where they were. I needed to look within.

Maybe I had left much of my self-confidence behind at Tulane. But I was now back to reclaim it. The steps I needed to take to steady my capsizing life began taking shape and started with the statement "Act as if you cannot fail."

Other ideas popped into my head.

Accept Full Responsibility for Your Actions

That's right—full responsibility. In reviewing my life, I had received some good breaks and some bad, just like everyone else. Part of my current career dilemma stemmed from having to start all over in establishing a law practice. I thought about the day I announced I was leaving my law firm to go work for a large company. A senior partner in the law firm urged me to reconsider leaving private practice. He counseled that clients were the foundation of a lawyer's career and allowed lawyers to control their own destiny. I had already shown early promise in business development, and by accepting a corporate position with one employer, I could be placing my entire career at its whim. It was the most profound and unfortunately the most prophetic career advice that I ever received. Marketing skills and the "ownership" of clients are much more critical to success than simply performing your job. Why do you think top salesmen are paid so well? Unfortunately, I didn't heed his advice at the time and placed my career in the hands of a large company, just as corporate America began turning on its employees.

Forget Regret or Life Is Yours to Miss

I remembered this line from the award-winning Broadway musical *Rent*. I had seen the phenomenal production several times, both on and off Broadway, and had practically memorized its soundtrack.

It was simply too late to look back now. I really can't say that I regretted working for the company. My stint there provided some valuable experience that I couldn't have otherwise obtained. Things often happen for a reason. You learn your lesson and then you need to move on.

It was definitely time for *me* to move on. But I wasn't sure what to do. Did I really need to start all over again? I couldn't exactly rewind my life to the beginning, even though this enticing but impossible notion plagued my thinking. Too often I had allowed past regret to ruin the present and cloud the future. If only I had done this or if only I had done that. Why did I invest in this stock? Why didn't I take that opportunity? If only . . . No! I needed to make a stand right here and right now and do the best I could with what I had. And even as hard as I could be on myself, I needed to realize and be grateful for my blessings, which included my health, education, and experience. I could either lament lost opportunities or reenergize and refocus my life along a path of rejuvenation and renewal. What I really needed at this midpoint of my life was a tune-up.

Midlife Tune-Up

I liked the automobile analogy. Over the years, I had come to realize the benefits of buying quality cars and driving them for a long time. My first new car right out of law school was an upscale sports car. It was more expensive than a "practical" car and most of my friends thought that I had splurged unnecessarily. But they were surprised when I kept driving the car year after year, and it looked just as good as the day I bought it. Many of them were already on their second or third cars by this time and had ended up spending just as much money, if not more, on their transportation needs. And I really enjoyed that car.

The automobile industry has undergone profound changes since the 1980s. Cars that used to peter out after 60,000 miles now run for hundreds of thousands of miles. My next automobile ran for over 200,000 miles and most people thought it was new. The car had 45,000 miles when I considered buying it and I was a concerned about the mileage. I brought it to be examined by my trusty mechanic before finalizing any purchase. He pointed at two similar models in his shop at the time and rattled off their mileage, 180,000 miles and 240,000 miles. He assured me, "This car is just getting broken in." He was right. And the automobile looked good and drove well because I kept it tuned up and in good repair.

Like automobiles, human life spans have been extended in both the quantity of years as well as the quality of life. Many of us are just hitting our stride or getting "broken in" at midlife. Our performance potential has now been extended by decades. Like quality cars, our bodies can also look good and drive well for a long time, provided that we focus on taking care of ourselves as opposed to being preoccupied by our odometers.

The Midlife Tune-Up Process

Once begun, a task is easy; half the work is done.
—Horace, *Epistles*

I reflected for some time on a process to tune up my own

life. Instead of changing sparks and plugs, it involved changing attitudes, outlook, and behavior. I had immersed myself in self-help literature for over twenty years and had attended many motivational seminars and retreats. I had also observed many happy and successful people. I eventually developed the six steps of the tune-up process, which all began with the letter *P.*

Passion. Passion is the seed of success and has been the basis of any significant achievement in my life. I had been very passionate about completing my education. Although my school days had been extremely hectic, they had also been good. During that challenging time, I was engaged in my quest, and my entire life sparked with vitality and energy. It was only later that my passion had waned. What things in your life are you truly passionate about? What gets you up in the morning? It is much easier and more enjoyable to pursue a path of passion.

Purpose. While I was a student, my purpose was crystal clear: getting through school. Once this goal was obtained, I often had trouble defining my next real purpose. Your purpose is what your life is directed towards. Once you find it, your life can explode into action. There is no better feeling than knowing in your heart that you are following your purpose and living the life you are meant to.

Power. Empowering yourself is one of the most important ideas in self-improvement. Power involves developing the unwavering confidence in yourself that you can in fact accomplish your purpose. I felt quite empowered in my quest to finish school, and that is why I did.

Planning. We perform at our best with clear, defined goals. With its institutional structure of assignments and semesters, school imposes its own planning scheme to organize your time around. But life does not always provide a syllabus, as well as graded and defined measures of progress. A critical discipline is to establish your own priorities and manage your own progress, instead of having it done for you. Remember to plan your work and then work your plan.

Perspective. Practically every self-help book I have ever read extols the virtues of having a proper perspective or a good attitude. Their constant refrain of the virtues of a positive attitude often reminds me of the hit tune that contemporary radio stations feel obliged to run into the ground. However, there is a good reason for emphasizing a healthy and optimistic outlook, for it does dramatically affect your quality of life and your ability to deal with the "slings and arrows of outrageous fortune."

Perseverance. The final tune-up step is perseverance. Nothing great was ever accomplished without overcoming tremendous obstacles and setbacks. Tragically, many people allow themselves to be deterred by various detours and bumps in the road, often when success is just around the corner. I once tried to inspire a friend who was experiencing similar hardships in completing his education. He wondered why I hadn't given up along the way. I replied that I had actually given up quite a few times. I just didn't quit.

Balancing the Tune-Up

All work and no play makes Jack a dull boy.
—Anonymous

Balance is a necessary ingredient of any self-improvement process. As you may have gathered from my story, I had been almost obsessively focused on my career at the expense of the other important areas of my life. I had driven myself to the point of exhaustion, passed on having a wife or family, and constantly denied myself life's simple pleasures. But I had little to show for all of my frenzied activity.

As I reflected on balance, I reviewed my notes from a spiritual retreat I had attended at the Manresa House of Retreats in Convent, Louisiana. My annual retreat at Manresa has become a significant part of my spiritual grounding. The facility has a national reputation and serves as the beautiful setting for three-day silent retreats, which allow participants time for rest and reflection. My most recent retreat master had been exceptional and had lectured on the benefits of leading a balanced life. He had illustrated his point with the cross of life:

Work: Approach work with pride but don't be consumed by it.

Play: Set aside time for play, be refreshed, and enjoy why you are working.

Worship: Acknowledge someone greater than ourselves.

Love: Be willing to sacrifice to make someone else happy.

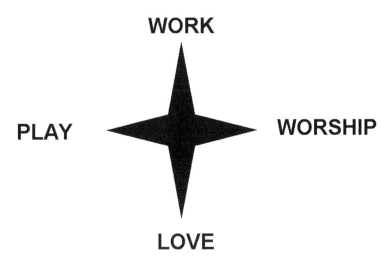

WORK

PLAY — WORSHIP

LOVE

Although the reasons for keeping your life in balance are simple, the practice can be difficult. For example, if you spend all your time making money and neglect your family and the other areas of your life, you are not going to have much to live for. The flip side is that if you spend all your time with your family and don't work, you are not going to be able to provide for them. We all need to maintain balance in our lives to avoid eventually toppling over. The important areas of life include emotional, financial, career, relationships, physical, mental, and spiritual.

Tuning Up Your Own Life

> Many receive advice, few profit by it.
> —Publilius Syrus, *Moral Sayings*

The principles in this book worked for me and I am confident that they will work for you. I am not saying that I have all the answers to all the questions. Anyone who claims that is probably exaggerating. What I am offering you is solid advice based upon my life experience, research, and insight.

I mentioned earlier that I have been a devoted reader of self-improvement literature for over twenty years, as much out of desperation as inspiration. I have expended considerable effort to find the answers in my own life, including seminars, retreats, self-help groups, and prayers. I have spent time meditating on the beautiful red rocks of Sedona, Arizona

and even sat in a sweat box for five hours a day for two weeks
trying to purify my mind and body. By the way, I enjoyed
Sedona much more than the sweat box. I have sat on more
than one counselor's couch and have solicited advice from
many successful people.

Most of the success principles contained in this book are
actually common sense. It doesn't take a rocket scientist to
figure out success. However, it does take a systematic
approach to be able to convert this common sense into the
insights and practices that can dramatically improve the
quality of your life.

The great challenge in any self-improvement program is
execution. If not implemented, such a program will fall by the
wayside as easily as do many perennial New Year's resolutions.
How many times have we been charged up by some motivational speaker or seminar only to quietly slip back into our
own mediocre routine? Consequently, I have presented this
book as a blueprint for improving your own life and organized it in a way that can be easily implemented as well as
understood. I have included a Tune-Up Plan Guide in
Appendix A and a suggested reading list in Appendix B to
assist you with your own tune-up process.

I can honestly say that the tune-up process dramatically
improved my own life. Within ninety days of applying the
principles, my life started to turn around significantly. I
took a chance, switched jobs, and attacked my career with
a renewed focus and vigor. I started an exercise and diet
program that helped me shed twenty-five pounds and feel
better physically than I had in years. I began meditating
each morning and felt a new calmness as I faced the day. I
dusted myself off from my stock-market losses, changed
financial advisers, and established my own plan for financial
independence. I began addressing some emotional issues
that had imprisoned me for many years. And I worked up
the courage to ask someone out to whom I was really
attracted. I became quickly smitten and for the first time
embraced rather than ran from intimacy and began to
make plans (albeit a little belatedly) to settle down and
start a family. I felt happier and more alive than I'd felt in
decades. I also began this book. I'd written several books,
two of which had been published. But this was the first

time that I was genuinely writing from my soul, and the feeling was exhilarating.

So, happy reading, and I sincerely hope that this book helps you tune up your own life into a great one.

CHAPTER 2

Challenges and Opportunities
of Midlife

Setting a good example for your children takes all the fun
out of middle age.

—William Feather, *The Business of Life*

There's only now;
There's only here.
Give in to love
Or live in fear.
No other path,
No other way,
No day but today.

—Jonathan Larson, *Rent*

What Is Midlife?

Since this book is entitled *Midlife Tune-Up*, it might be useful to try to grapple with that elusive term, *midlife*. Does it
necessarily start at forty, the time that unflattering birthday
cards start showing up at your home? Or is midlife even
younger, the fateful day when someone calls you "ma'am" or
"sir" or when a particular birthday somehow strikes you
between the eyes? Many consider their thirtieth birthday a
rite of passage from being "young." I did at the time,
although thirty seems mighty young these days.

But *midlife*, like so many things, is a relative term, particularly in our rapidly changing society. It is hard to believe
that, at the turn of the previous century, the average life
span was in the midforties. However, the past century witnessed dramatic medical advances as well as awareness and
changes in lifestyle, which have served to nearly double
the average life span to what we enjoy today. In addition,
society's attitude about aging has changed. The baby
boomers, in particular, are taking better care of themselves

and constructively addressing the aging process. They generally perceive themselves as much younger for their age than their parents did. The Web site psychologytoday.com defines *midlife transition* as a normal process of maturing that occurs to many of us at about age forty, give or take twenty years. Midlife can be a moving target. Today's fifty is yesterday's forty.

If one approaches the question of midlife from a purely quantitative standpoint, then the middle portion of an average life span of eighty years would range from the age twenty-seven to age fifty-five. However, I don't know many twenty-seven-year-olds who would appreciate being told that they are entering midlife. In addition, many fifty-five-year-olds, despite their AARP cards, do not consider themselves old. And they shouldn't.

One broad grouping of midlifers would be today's baby boomers. That group is defined by the media and sociologists as those born between (and including) 1946 and 1964. Most baby boomers were deeply affected by the events, music, and social changes of the 1960s. It was the baby boomers who pushed the divorce rates to 50 percent.

But let's not dwell on age. As a society we are too obsessed with the chronological number in measuring the aging process, which put less technically means how old you are. In his classic book *Ageless Body, Timeless Mind,* noted author Deepak Chopra quite insightfully outlined three measures for age. The first, of course, is one's chronological age. However, Chopra points out that one's physical condition is another very important way to measure one's age. Both appearance and physical vigor can vary dramatically with age. How good do you look and feel for your age? We all know people who look either much younger or older than they actually are.

Another measure of age is one's emotional age. How good or how young do you *feel* on the inside? One's emotional state of mind is very important to one's well-being. I know some people in their seventies and eighties who are emotionally younger than people half their age. Their eyes sparkle brightly and they dive into life and relish every aspect. My grandmother was one of those people. She never seemed old, even while she was in her nineties.

The point is that one's chronological age (how old you are)

generally has less impact on your well-being than do your physical or emotional age. Yet it is obsessively focused on. In a book entitled *Age Wave*, author Ken Dychtwald discusses the impact of longevity on our population. On a recent "60 Minutes" appearance, he chronicled the development of many people in their seventies and eighties returning to the workplace. Don't tell them to hang it up after fifty-five. Many at this stage have as much as thirty years left in second and third careers. If you approach midlife properly, you can ensure that the second half of life is even better than the first. To begin with, you generally have more control over it.

My grandmother, my Momie, lived until the age of ninety-nine and stood as a vivid example in my life of defying the aging process. She was very active until her death and more importantly was decades younger, both emotionally and physically, than her years. Although she was widowed in her fifties, she didn't stop living and resign herself to following her husband to the grave after a few years. Instead, she moved in with my family and enjoyed another forty years of quality life, a good portion of which was devoted to helping my mother raise my younger sister and me. Although she was fortunate to have two good daughters (including my mother) and understanding sons-in-law to take care of her, she gave back significantly. She was an extremely important person in my life and often my only refuge in a tumultuous household that experienced its share of domestic discord, financial stress, and substance abuse. She kept herself young with her children and grandchildren and eventually great-grandchildren and great-great-grandchildren.

She also loved to gamble. I remember my mother bringing her to various ladies' houses three or four nights a week to play cards. A few years after I graduated from law school, my grandmother went to live with my aunt and uncle in Mobile. For her eighty-sixth birthday, the family took her to Las Vegas. She arrived that morning with my aunt and uncle and I came later that night. When I entered the hotel lobby of the Riviera, the first thing I noticed was my grandmother sitting forlorn on a couch by the registration desk. I became disturbed, thinking that something truly bad had happened. My aunt explained that she had lost all of her money in the first day of gambling, including the complimentary markers supplied by the casino. However, she rallied when she saw me and gave me my first tour of a Las Vegas casino. Her eyes blazed with excitement as she stood amongst the swirl of lights and sounds. "Isn't this wonderful?" she exclaimed.

A few years later she moved to Las Vegas with my aunt and uncle. I would visit regularly and she loved to introduce me to the dealers, who all knew her. She would always dress immaculately and liked to wear attractive pins.

She would also visit during the holidays. On one such visit, Christmas day, she fell and broke her hip. At the time, she was ninety-three years old. The irony was that there were no fewer than a dozen family members standing around when she fell, including me. But not one of us was able to break her fall. A nice holiday turned to horror as we waited for the ambulance with my grandmother in such obvious pain.

The next day, Momie was operated on and the doctors reported that the surgery was successful. However, they could make no promises about whether she would ever walk again. The next few days were trying as Momie drifted in and out of consciousness. I put statues of angels around her room and played soothing music. By New Year's, Momie was becoming herself and she made some bets on the bowl games. She still had a long way to go, but she insisted to everyone, including the hospital personnel, that she was going back to Las Vegas.

She seemed the only one not surprised when thirty days later she boarded a plane to Las Vegas with the help only of a walker. While her doctors were astonished, I knew the true reason for her rapid recovery. She wanted to get back to the blackjack table.

Her passion for her family and for gambling kept her young and helped her recover from a serious injury. Despite her advancing years, she never seemed old.

So *midlife* is a relative term. Some people are more comfortable with it than others. For purposes of this book, midlife is sometime after you enter the workforce (which includes running a household) on a full-time basis and before you retire from full-time work.

Challenges of Midlife

What could be more enchanting than a dear, old lady growing wise with age? Every age can be enchanting provided you live within it.

—Brigitte Bardot

Always fall in with what you're asked to accept. Take what is given, and make it over your way. My aim in life has always been to hold my own with whatever's going. Not against; with.

—Robert Frost

What a drag it is getting old.

—Mick Jagger and Keith Richards,
"Mother's Little Helper"

Midlife can present many challenges, particularly in a society obsessed with youth and beauty. We are constantly bombarded by messages from the media, usually from those wanting to sell us something, that we are generally not good enough on our own and need their products for better and more fulfilling lives. In particular, we are barraged by the recurring theme that old is bad and young is good and we need to do everything possible to look, feel, and act young. Some of the specific challenges of midlife include:

- Fear of the aging process, primarily the physical changes to your body.
- Alarm that the best part of your life is behind you and that you have little to look forward to.
- Regret over paths taken or not taken, such as the choice of a particular career or spouse, and disappointment over not having achieved the dreams of your youth.

Fear of Aging

The greeting-card industry has perpetuated this obsession with age. Any card for a birthday past the age of twenty-nine is invariably black and portrays its recipient as a depreciating asset that is less valuable and less functional than just a day earlier. Phrases such as *over the hill* are quite typical, particularly once we reach "the big four-oh." Such cards seem more to memorialize one's passing than celebrate one's living.

Although meant in fun, these cards send powerful messages that aging is bad, something to be avoided or ashamed about. It is unfortunate that our society places so much value on youth and beauty. The American culture is one of the few to have this obsession. In many other cultures that are less appearance oriented, aging is not viewed so negatively. The elders are respected instead of shunted off.

Who can forget the dramatic scene from the classic movie *The Wizard of Oz* where Dorothy is locked up in a room by the Wicked Witch of the West? The witch then turns over the hourglass and shouts to a terrified Dorothy that this is how long she has left to live (although we're never quite sure what is actually intended for Dorothy). We all remember the horror in Dorothy's eyes as her friends, the Scarecrow, the Tin Man, and the Cowardly Lion, all try to break down the door before the hourglass runs out.

Many of us are likewise fixated on the hourglass of our own lives. We torment ourselves by focusing on the time slithering away and piling up at the bottom of our hourglass instead of living in the present. Although the hourglass is a telling reminder that life is precious and finite, it doesn't necessarily mean that our quality of life will decrease.

A tune-up can help you enjoy the rest of your life. How much better could you feel physically? Imagine yourself financially independent or in a career that you loved. Remember that you are not Dorothy and there is no Wicked Witch, so forget the hourglass.

Of course, the reality is that our bodies do age. We are simply not going to look the same as we did when we were younger. But it is still possible to remain attractive and even beautiful as we mature. It is so refreshing to see a whole generation of mature movie stars defy the conventional wisdom about show business and aging. Such stars include Sophia Loren, Susan Sarandon, Cher, Goldie Hawn, and Sela Ward. On the male side we have the timeless Sean Connery. Who said James Bond was washed up after he got a little paunchy and lost his hair? Sean Connery is more popular now than he ever was. John Travolta reinvented himself in his forties in the movie *Pulp Fiction*. Even rock stars can age well, with Sting and Jon Bon Jovi enjoying success as sex symbols and entertainers in middle age.

You might argue that these entertainers have more access to cosmetics, nutritionists, physical trainers, and cosmetic surgery. And you're probably correct. But anti-aging products, services, and procedures are becoming more available and acceptable. However, you don't want to go overboard.

The point is not to look as if you're twenty again but to look good for your age. My grandmother was a lovely woman in her nineties. She always dressed impeccably and was complimented wherever she went. I often took her to casinos and people were always fascinated with her. Obviously, no one would have mistaken her for a young woman, but she looked decades younger, as she matured very gracefully. And she never had a lick of surgery. My mother also looks outstanding for her age.

As the slogan goes, don't lie about your age . . . defy it. The idea is to look good for your age but not try to be a teenager again.

"My Best Years Are Behind Me"

> People are like wine—some turn to vinegar, but the best improve with age.
>
> —Pope John XXIII

I have heard "my best years are behind me" from friends far too many times. In some cases, people lament giving their "best years" to their former spouses: "I gave him/her the best years of my life!" But how does anyone know for sure what their best years are before their life has finished? Are they simply assuming that their younger years are better because they are supposed to be? After all, you're "young" then.

But who is to say that your teens and twenties are necessarily your best years, particularly in a society where kids are growing up much too fast? Or even that your thirties were your best years? As I write this book, I firmly believe that my best years are still ahead. My earlier years were times of tremendous pain and growth. I feel fortunate to have survived considerable turmoil and self-destructive tendencies. Today, I am more content, having conquered many of my demons, than I have been in some time. More importantly, I'm looking forward to the future as I steer my life and plan those activities that offer me the most fulfillment. I anticipate the opportunities ahead as opposed to lamenting the years behind.

Would you really want to be twenty years old again? Think

of all the struggles between then and now. Think of all the learning experiences, some quite painful, that you were forced to deal with. Would you really want all that pain and ignorance back? If I have any regret, it is that I did not enjoy my past years enough. I always seemed to be more focused on what I wanted rather than what I had, more worried about the mountains ahead instead of the hills behind (how many mountains in your life turn out to be hills?). I was too preoccupied with my problems as opposed to my gifts, the people who irritated me rather than the ones who loved me, the opportunities I missed out on rather than the goals I achieved, and so on. But those years taught me something, to live.

Regret and Disappointment

There is an old saying that you will get in a wreck if you drive while looking in the rearview mirror. This attitude of urgency in living is legitimate. Don't wait until you have a brush with death or a friend or loved one passes away to suddenly realize that you need to live. A vivid example of living in the present is Jonathan Larson, the critically acclaimed author of the Pulitzer Prize-winning *Rent*. Producing a play on Broadway is a monumentally difficult task. First there is the composition of the musical and the integration of the story line, music, and choreography to create what many believe to be the most memorable entertainment experiences available. Even after a Broadway musical is written, there are still the immense challenges of financing and producing it. Larson had successfully achieved all these goals, but the tragedy is that he died suddenly at the age of thirty-six, the same day that *Rent* opened on Broadway to tremendous acclaim. His biography on the playbill for *Rent* reminds us all to live in the present.

Jonathan Larson was intensely passionate about living life, creating music and changing his part of the world—Broadway musical theater. The exuberance, the passion and philosophy of *Rent* are clear reflections of his life and the way he chose to live it. Jonathan's sudden, unexpected death on the very day his dream came true is a sobering reminder to make the most of the time we have. Listen to his music, reach out to your community, and celebrate all the love in your life. No day but today.

Part of resolving regret involves letting go of the past. If you found you have been overburdened by work or distracted by worry, then resolve to make the necessary changes in your life. Begin enjoying each day and accepting yourself. There is a fine line between self-acceptance and self-improvement. Although goal setting is an important part of the tune-up process, it should not be at the expense of your peace of mind and well-being. Plan for the future, but live in the present. Don't lament your imperfections; just try to continually improve yourself. Avoid the polar extremes of the self-improvement continuum—stagnation versus chaos.

Stagnation involves surrendering to the status quo, ignoring those areas of your life with which you are not completely satisfied. As humans, we are inherently imperfect and there is much about us that can be improved. We all have bad habits and tendencies that prevent us from living a more fulfilling life but that we often are reluctant to address. Stagnation involves settling into a comfort zone that resists change. Self-improvement requires the discipline, focus, and courage to make necessary changes. Such positive steps could include starting an exercise program or making an appointment with a financial planner. Rather than becoming mired in regret over the past, focus on the desired changes in your life today and plan ahead.

At the other extreme, chaos involves constant struggle and striving, torturing ourselves with a negative litany of self-talk in which we berate ourselves and our choices. Our minds taunt us with streams of images of how things could or should have been. Regret consumes us and we find ourselves immersed in negativity, sometimes flailing about erratically, struggling to piece our lives together. Such frantic efforts often sink us even deeper and make us vulnerable to unhealthy diversions such as substance abuse or illicit affairs to provide relief.

The happy medium is to accept your mistakes, to understand that life is a learning process and that the people and events of your past were all placed there to teach you important lessons. Your challenge today is whether or not you will learn from the past and plan for a better, more productive future or be paralyzed by regret or drift along, prone to the same errors as before. Whenever I would complain to a friend about my catastrophe du jour, she would ask, "What lesson did you learn?" I found that when I focused on the lessons, I was less prone to make more mistakes and to regret the past.

We all have regrets over choices made or not made. Perhaps your marriage or relationship didn't work out or your career stalled out or you were not as financially success-ful as you had dreamed. If you remember, I was moping about all three.

But all is not lost. There is always time to change and regroup. That applies to marriages as well as careers. Nothing gave me more pleasure than to see my mother remarry in her fifties after enduring nearly three decades with my father. I don't want to speak badly about my father, as he recently passed away after a valiant fight with cancer. I cared for him during his illness and fortunately was able to reestablish our relationship. However, my father was not the best husband, preferring the company of his drinking buddies to his wife and treating her as somewhat of an afterthought in his life. He was never physically abusive; he simply wasn't there physically. As his drinking progressed, his career declined and we always seemed just a few steps ahead of his creditors.

When I tried to talk my mother into finally leaving him, she initially balked. I had recognized their marriage as an empty shell for years, but she still wanted to hold on for some reason. I asked her why and she replied "the companionship." I asked her when was the last time the two of them had gone any-where together. She couldn't remember. I then asked when was the last time they had really even sat down and talked. She couldn't remember that either. I told her that, in reality, she had no companion and hadn't had one for years.

When she finally did leave him, she became deeply depressed. Although their split and the subsequent sale of our heavily mortgaged house had relieved her and myself (I had guaranteed the mortgage at one point to save the house from foreclosure) of his considerable financial problems, she was very despondent. Having worked only sporadically over the years, she was worried about her financial future. I promised her that she would never have to live in uncomfortable conditions. To reinforce my promise, I rented a nice house into which my mother, my grandmother, and I moved together.

My mother was also worried about companionship. Who would possibly want her at her age? She was in her early fifties, and I found myself in the strange role of counseling my mother about dating. At that time, I was in my late twenties and was never particularly wild about the singles scene myself. I cringed at the thought of my mother being "out there." She was from the old school and I fretted that she was about to enter a world that she could not imagine. But at least she had the courage to go "out there." She joined a singles club and began attending social events for people in her age group. I told her to just go and have a good time and I would wait up to see how she made out. I had braced myself for perhaps a long stint in my new role as head of household.

How shocked I was when she suddenly started dating a very nice gentleman who was taking her to more places in a few weeks than my father had in the last ten years. Then just before Christmas, I returned home from my office party and they arrived shortly afterwards, giddy as teenagers, with my mother sporting an engagement ring. He had come to ask me for her hand in marriage. He turned out to be a wonderful husband and they had a great marriage. He became a tremendous asset to our family and I loved him as my own father.

Tragically, he died recently, but not before giving my mother seventeen great years. And I'm proud to say that my mother never wavered through the tragedy, caring for him heroically and bearing her enormous loss with dignity and valor. But after his death, she didn't sit at home and feel sorry for herself at the age of seventy-two. She became active in social activities, shook off breast cancer (she is in complete remission), and actually started dating again.

Life can provide other chances, but you have to give life the opportunity. If you have missed something on the first go-round, it is not too late on the second or even the third one. My mother is a good example of that.

Remember that it is never too late to achieve your dreams.

But you need to focus on the opportunities available.

Opportunities of Midlife

> I don't think of all the misery, but of the beauty that still remains. . . . My advice is: Go outside, to the fields, enjoy nature and the sunshine, go out and try to recapture happiness in yourself and in God. Think of all the beauty that's still left in and around you and be happy!
>
> —Anne Frank

If you want to change your life, you have to give life the opportunity. This requires that you assess your situation and muster the courage to change. If you have dreams, it is never too late to turn them into reality. But first you need the courage to try.

Many people have made dramatic changes at midlife when they could have easily accepted the status quo. Do you recognize the following person who made quite a change in his life?

He started his career as a radio announcer and then eventually became a screen actor, actually starring in some popular movies. However, in his midforties, his career began to wane and he was reduced to taking less flattering roles. To make matters worse, his marriage began to sour at this time. His wife had just won an Academy Award and decided she was destined for bigger and better things, which did not include him. Her career was rising and his was going the other way. So she left him.

There he was at midlife, with seemingly no place to go. However, out of the ashes of his failed marriage and stalled acting career came a burning desire to enter politics. He became fascinated with the political theater and quickly understood the emerging impact of television on the political process. He became a spokesman for General Electric, which allowed him to tour the country, giving speeches and refining his method. He later attracted notice with an eloquent keynote address at a nationally televised political convention. But still no one took him seriously when he decided to run for governor of California against a popular incumbent, who had beaten no less than former vice-president and then eventual president Richard Nixon in the previous election. Although the former actor had little experience with the complex issues necessary to run a state, particularly one that size, he recognized that his communication skills could be used quite effectively as a citizen-politician challenging the status quo. He finally convinced a prominent political consultant in California to help this politically inexperienced actor take on the formidable incumbent. The consulting firm summarized all of the issues to be addressed in the race into 100 index cards, which the actor then memorized. He ad-libbed the rest. Still no one gave him much of a chance.

But the conventional political wisdom was turned on its head when the actor's communication skills struck a chord with the average voter. At the age of fifty-five, Ronald Reagan started his new career in politics by being elected governor of California by a margin of 1 million votes.

Although still not taken seriously on a national level, Ronald Reagan persisted and at the age seventy was elected president of the United States. Whether you like him or not, Reagan had a profound impact on the office of president. The man that he defeated, Jimmy Carter, had suffered through a difficult presidency despite having his party in the majority in both the House and the Senate. Previous presidents like Nixon and Johnson had been labeled as failures also. Some political scholars were even questioning the office of president, and a book at that time entitled *Twilight of the Presidency* argued that the office had lost its constitutional effectiveness. However, Ronald Reagan redefined the office of the modern president, and subsequent presidencies, including those of the Bushes and Bill Clinton, were modeled after that of "the Gipper." Ronald Reagan also redefined what it means to be a senior citizen, proving that one can be very effective and optimistic even in one's senior years. When Reagan's age became an issue in the second campaign, he was able to scoff at it with one of the most memorable lines in political debates, claiming that he "would not take advantage" of his opponent's "youth and inexperience."

So think about Ronald Reagan the next time you think that your dreams have passed you by. He could have easily decided to retire quietly rather than plunge so heartily into his new career.

Too many of us approach middle age with the idea that life has somehow passed us by, that some of the great dreams we had as youths have dissipated and we will never be able to realize them. We look enviously at others and wonder about the source of their success. If only we could have known then what we know now, we think. But the fact is that we know it now and many people do not hit their stride until midlife. And there are advantages to having success come a little later in life.

How classic are the woeful tales of rock stars or athletes who have 95 percent of their earning capacity squeezed into a few young years but then end up jobless and destitute later in life? In many cases, they were unable to adjust to their megasuccess because it occurred before they were mature enough to handle it. Many simply didn't have the life experience to deal with the fame and fortune that came knocking at their door—and often ended up knocking them over. We all know of the Michael Jordans and the John Elways who turn lucrative sports careers into endorsements or other business ventures, but many more athletes squander their funds and their opportunities. And the number of rock stars who ease into retirement is even lower. Many have to continually tour (usually playing to much smaller audiences) just to make a living.

One athlete who went against the grain was Magic Johnson. When he was thirty-two years old, the Los Angeles Lakers star basketball player had an extreme reversal of fortunes. As you know, Johnson made national headlines when he tested positive for the AIDS virus. Not only did he have to retire from basketball, the career that he loved, but his death seemed imminent. Losing your career and possibly your life is a midlife crisis any way you cut it. Overnight he went from being young, successful, and envied to being a tragic figure, maybe even facing the end of his life. But Magic Johnson persevered against his illness and today is disease free. In addition, his business career has soared and he has stood tall as a visible symbol in the prevention of the dreaded AIDS virus. Magic Johnson is an example not only of great emotional resiliency but also a reminder that life is precious and each day must be cherished.

J. K. Rowling, the author of the wildly popular Harry Potter series of books, was a struggling mother in her thirties who was abandoned and left to care for her infant child on her own. She was forced to go on welfare but wrote the book that launched her career in coffeehouses while her daughter slept in a stroller by her side. Just over a decade later, her fortune was estimated to be larger than the queen of England's.

Many others made their mark at midlife. At the age of fifty-two, a struggling milkshake-mixer salesman named Raymond Kroc was wondering how it could be that a little hamburger joint owned by two brothers in Southern California was his best customer. He couldn't figure out how this little upstart business could be ordering so many machines, while business from his five-and-dime and corner drugstore customers kept declining. Kroc, a high-school dropout who once played the piano in bordellos and speakeasies, boarded a plane from his home in Chicago to meet the owners in California. He returned as the national franchising agent for McDonald's.

Within a year, in 1955, he poured all of his resources into opening the first outlet in suburban Chicago that would become Kroc's prototype for turning burgers and fries into a mass-market empire. The store, a red-and-white-tiled box with a neon yellow arch on each side, boasted a small menu featuring a fifteen-cent hamburger. Within ten years, McDonald's would have more than 700 sites and by 2003 would have 31,100 outlets in 119 countries, feeding 47 million people every day, with annual sales of $17.1 billion.

Kentucky Fried Chicken was started by Colonel Sanders when he was in his sixties. At the time, his only asset was a chicken recipe. He went around to many stores trying to sell it and received nearly a thousand nos before he received his first yes.

Another good example of success as a midlife restaurateur is Ruth Fertel, who hailed from my hometown of New Orleans. All of her friends wondered why a middle-aged divorced mother, who had no experience in the food-service business, would purchase a struggling restaurant in New Orleans named Chris's Steak House. She brought her own touch to the establishment, renaming it to Ruth's Chris Steak House as well as making some important changes to its operations. She ordered the highest-quality meat and then cooked the steaks so sizzling hot that a distinctive hiss could be heard when the plates were presented. She was very successful, expanding and franchising outlets throughout the country. Recently, Ruth's Chris went public.

As I stated earlier, many people don't hit their stride until middle age. In some cases, it wasn't until the second and even third career that a person really made a mark. The man whom Ronald Reagan defeated, Jimmy Carter, arguably enjoyed his peak moment after the presidency, when he received the Nobel Peace Prize. Despite his crushing presidential defeat, Carter reinvented himself after the White House, when many others might have chosen to fade into the sunset. Many now consider Carter one of the most successful former presidents.

And, of course, the ultimate comeback kid is Abraham Lincoln. Although self-help books regularly feature this remarkable individual, his life puts failure and disappointment into proper perspective. Consider his biography:

> Mother died: Age ten
> Failed in business: Age twenty-two
> Defeated for legislature: Age twenty-three
> Passed over for federal appointment: Age thirty-nine
> Defeated for U.S. Congress: Age forty-five
> Defeated for U.S. Senate: Age forty-six
> Lost vice-presidency of the United States: Age forty-seven
> Elected president of the United States: Age fifty-one

Success is rarely an accident and has been defined as that time when preparation meets opportunity. The more life experience that you accumulate, the more likely it is that you will experience success, provided that you keep improving and preparing yourself. As Abraham Lincoln wrote in his diary, "I will study and prepare myself and one day my time will come." What a great thought! Even if you haven't achieved at the levels that you think you can, it is never too late. The good news is that the seeming challenges of midlife are also accompanied by opportunities.

Although there will always be the proverbial computer whiz kids, such as Bill Gates and Michael Dell, who amassed considerable wealth when they were very young, it is usually the midyears when your greatest earning potential kicks in.

Challenge of Assessing

> If a person is to get the meaning of life he must learn to like the facts about himself—ugly as they may seem to his sentimental vanity—before he can learn the truth behind the facts. And the truth is never ugly.
>
> —Eugene O'Neill

An effective midlife tune-up requires complete honesty in assessing your life. It is amazing what hoops people will jump through to avoid being truthful with themselves. Honesty implies a totally unbiased view of your life. How many of us stay in relationships or jobs that we are not happy with? We try to convince ourselves that things are working when they are really not. Do you have a solid financial plan, or do you simply hope that sufficient resources will be there when you decide to retire? What about your health? We are all aware of the benefits of proper diet and exercise. But for some reason, we keep putting it off. We might weigh a little more than we would like, but we avoid confirming this with a scale and setting a plan to reach a desirable weight.

Although it might be painful, be absolutely honest with yourself in assessing your life. Many of us want to varnish the truth for some reason and gloss over our rough spots. If you are sincere about self-improvement, examine your life honestly as you work through the tune-up process. One of the most exciting things about our society is the ability to make positive changes in our lives. It is never too late to change your life around, provided that you are sincere in your efforts. There are many people out there who overcame enormous obstacles, including serious illness and handicaps, to lead happy, productive lives. We intuitively know the truth about ourselves. Once we can admit this truth, we can start down our path to positive change.

There are several common attributes in those who succeed, which I have incorporated in my tune-up process. Successful people had a defined purpose about which they were passionate. They empowered themselves despite any obstacles. They had perspective, they planned, and, most of all, they persevered. Think of Abraham Lincoln. No one becomes one of our greatest presidents without being able to overcome enormous setbacks.

PART 2

The Tune-Up Proce

CHAPTER 3

Overview of the Six Simple Steps

First say to yourself what you would be; and then do what you have to do.

—Epictetus, *Discourses*

What you can do or dream you can, begin it.
Boldness has genius, power, and magic in it.

—Goethe

In the previous chapter, we discussed the opportunities and pitfalls of midlife. Such a time can bring on what is commonly known as a midlife crisis. The primary goal of this book is to transform your midlife crisis into midlife *clarity,* through the tune-up process. The tune-up process involves systematically examining and evaluating the important areas of your life and redirecting each area towards meaningful outcomes, while still living fully and enjoying yourself.

Many reach midlife with the grim feeling of being stuck—trapped in a marriage, career, or situation over which they have little control. We feel immobilized and helpless. But the laws of physics tell us that items at rest tend to stay at rest, but items in motion tend to move ahead. The best way to extricate yourself from any situation is to simply get going, move out of your rut, and work the tune-up steps.

The tune-up process can also be considered a period of renewal:

Renewing yourself
Renewing your passions
Renewing your commitment
Renewing your drive
Renewing your focus

This process requires examining your life to determine the parts that are working and the parts that are not. The tune-up process provides you with a framework for such self-examination. Self-renewal comes from your core. Don't depend on external circumstances or aspects of your life beyond your control to make you happy. You have to make a conscious decision to renew, which often involves detaching from old habits; letting go of past feelings, past guilt, past insecurities, and past doubts; and creating a new you.

This process can be painstaking. It involves constant effort and is not as easy as simply repeating, " I believe in myself," as some of the more superficial self-help books like to propose. If you have been plagued by doubts and insecurities, they are not going away overnight. Instead, commit to a careful and gradual transformation. As we will discuss, your personal relationships can be critical to your tune-up. It is often necessary to surround yourself with people who will support you and rid yourself of those who don't. Too often, friends and even family members can feel threatened by your desire to better yourself and can end up subtly sabotaging your efforts. If you find you have too many negative people around, then you need to make some changes.

Much of the tune-up or renewal process is accomplished on a subconscious or intuitive level, so one needs to allocate adequate "quiet time" to reflect and plan. This can often be difficult in a time when we are so addicted to stimulation. We seem to be overstimulated in every nook and cranny of our lives, and there is often little solitude in our networked world of computers, cell phones, beepers, BlackBerries, and other PDAs.

Self-renewal requires a total commitment. Many leave self-help seminars excited and saturated with energy and ideas. Others set lofty goals for themselves at year end. We may have the best of intentions, but it is usually not long before our regular habits kick in and we suddenly become too "busy" to work on our dreams. We lose sight of our goals and find it much easier to descend back into our familiar routines. The idea of change can be quite overwhelming. Sometimes we don't know where to start and therefore tend to procrastinate.

That is why I developed the tune-up process, which breaks

the task of self-renewal down into six simple steps that can be applied to all areas of your life. The key is to move past your inertia, commit to the tune-up, and start your renewal process. The six steps of the tune-up process, which we discussed in Part 1, are as follows:

1. Passion
2. Purpose
3. Power
4. Planning
5. Perspective
6. Perseverance

As I mentioned, I had spent over two decades immersed in the self-help world, constantly studying articles, books, and audiocassette tapes, analyzing performance strategies, as well as observing successful people. Some of my own lessons came easily, while others required considerable effort and sometimes heartache before eventually sinking in. The tune-up steps contain lessons learned through my own research, observation, and experience and provide a helpful method for organizing and implementing this life-changing process.

Each of the tune-up steps is important as well as interrelated. Together, they can integrate into an unstoppable synergy that can make your life soar. Consider how *passion* and *purpose* can work so powerfully together. Your *passion* can be fueled by discovering your *purpose*, an overriding goal in your life that you are wildly enthusiastic about. This enthusiasm about your *purpose* ignites your *passion*, which in turn drives you towards your *purpose*.

Conversely, the entire tune-up process can easily be sabotaged by neglecting a step, just like missing a rung as you climb a ladder can send you plunging downwards. For example, many people have a *purpose* for which they have tremendous *passion*, but they hesitate to pursue their vision or dreams because of fear or self-doubt. That is why *power* is so important, not in the sense of dominating others but rather of empowering yourself to pursue your goals. But even empowered, you're not going to make much progress without proper *planning*. There is a big myth in our society about "overnight" successes—those who hit it big, almost by accident. But such accidental successes tend to be the exception rather than the rule, and most successful people don't reach the top by chance. Any notable success is usually the result of years of careful *planning*. In addition, a proper *perspective* is indispensable during one's climb—maintaining the proper attitude, learning from your mistakes, and always keeping an eye on the big picture. Finally, successful people *persevere* during the rough times and setbacks, refusing to quit and pushing ahead in pursuit of the goals important to them.

The tune-up process can be an important way to energize and redirect your life. Some of the steps will be easier than others, and generally the steps we find most difficult are the ones that have hindered us in the past. I have already discussed my crisis with confidence and the need to re-empower myself so that I could more effectively pursue my goals. And it is not enough to simply focus on career goals. At one point in time, my life was so badly out of balance that I was sabotaging my cherished career goals without even knowing it. It is important to apply the tune-up process to all areas of your life—emotional, financial, career, relationship, physical, mental, and spiritual—so that you live a balanced and more fulfilling life. Hopefully, your journey will not be as long and arduous as mine.

CHAPTER 4

Step 1: Passion

Nothing great in the world has ever been accomplished without passion.

—Hegel, *Philosophy of History*

(n.) Strong enthusiastic liking for something; powerful, intense emotion; intensity of feeling or reaction.

Recover Your Passion

The tune-up process starts with recovering your passion for life. After we've experienced some defeats and disappointments, it is often easy for our passion to wane. We become disillusioned and disconnected, and we approach each day mechanically by getting up and going through the motions. We lose our zest for living, and our life gradually becomes one of endless drudgery as opposed to an exciting adventure.

There is an old saying that you start off life ready to conquer the world but then become content simply to own a piece of real estate. Then you spend your entire life trying to pay off that piece of real estate. At the end of life, you find yourself contained in a piece of real estate. What a dim and narrow view of the world! Why is it we all start off with lofty goals but then often become quickly disillusioned in the face of life's setbacks and adversities?

And if you dwell on it long enough, you can find plenty to be disillusioned about. Our world is no longer safe, and this is certainly a legitimate cause for concern. Our lives have become much more complicated and hectic. But there is also much to be grateful for. We still live in the most affluent society in the history of the world. Many are willing to risk their life savings as well their lives for the immense opportunity and privileges that can be found in the United States of America. So as long as your health is good, find something to be passionate about, and then get going. It is hard to find a successful person who is not passionate about something.

I remember myself charged up and ready to take on the world. Then as my own disappointments began to accumulate, I became increasingly disillusioned and more willing to "settle" in life. I resigned myself to simply getting by. But as I came to grips with my own listlessness, I knew that it was important to reignite my own passion and my purpose for living. I wanted to feel that same rush for living that I felt in my youth.

Reflecting on your youth can be a key to reigniting your passion. Think about that little voice inside you that whispered your dreams. Many of us had youthful goals or ideals that stirred our passion but that we never pursued. Such aspirations don't simply vanish but remain latent in our subconscious, gnawing at us from time to time. This can bring that unsettling feeling that we are not doing what we are supposed to do. Such remorse can sap our lives of passion.

I am reminded of a sad story of an acquaintance whose teenage daughter had a strong passion for ballet and was even accepted into a prestigious dance academy in New York. However, her family could not afford the tuition, and she was unable to attend. I don't want to criticize the family, which had modest means and several other children to support. Perhaps their decision to forego this once-in-a-lifetime opportunity for their daughter was simple economic reality. But the disappointment had a profound effect on the girl. She dropped out of college and became withdrawn and rebellious. She found herself in an unhealthy relationship with someone who was abusive and immature. Her mother confided all of this to me after the fact, and I wish I had known the family earlier. I knew a little bit about begging and borrowing my way through school and perhaps could have offered some advice. There may have been grants, scholarships, or loans available that could have prevented a young dream from being strangled.

We have all had similar disappointments in our youth. Although I always had a great passion for writing, I believe that it was short-circuited for a number of years by a creative writing class I took in college. Although the professor liked some of the work I had done, he seemed distant and condescending. I failed to receive my usual A in the class, and maybe the B was just enough to discourage me in this area.

I finally began writing again and even had some success in getting published. But I would quickly become disappointed when my book sales were not as strong as I expected. For a while, I stopped writing, as different things began to capture my attention. I felt myself draining away. I needed to start writing again. I became reenergized in writing this book. Writing and sharing ideas is what I'm passionate about. I can spend long hours at the computer screen and not even realize the time that has passed.

Passion is the fuel that energizes your soul. When you feel that you are pouring out your whole soul with what you do—whether it is fixing automobiles, cutting lawns, or any project—that is passion.

Rediscovering lost passion can take a bit of work as well as courage. Our egos can be quite fragile in our youth. How many times have some of your so-called "friends" poked fun at your lofty dreams, which you then quickly disclaimed? Unfortunately, people tend to resent the success of their peers. Parents also have a tendency to steer their children into traditional career paths. It is so important that parents help children to nurture their own passions rather than try to redirect them into "safer" occupations.

One of the challenges of midlife is to rediscover the passion of your youth—that same unbridled optimism that you had in your late teens and twenties, that belief that you could really make a difference in the world. The truth is you still can.

Passion is not just about career or financial goals; it cuts across all areas of your life. Passion is your joy for living. It goes beyond your dreams and aspirations but also involves connecting with that playful, pleasurable self that appreciates the simple wonders of life. I remember one evening after a horrendous day at work. I had worked late, as usual, had stopped off at a fast-food outlet for something quick to take home, as usual, and was a little irritated at having to wait, as usual. My mind was lost in my demanding day, and I wasn't in the best of moods as I waited for the hamburger that I intended to gobble down at home before diving into the pile of work that I had lugged with me. Apparently, I had made up my mind to cap off my difficult day with a miserable evening, and I was doing a very good job of it. But while I waited, I noticed a pinball machine in the restaurant. How long had it been since I had played pinball? I had loved pinball in my youth—the lights, the bells, the clanging as you battled to keep that the little silver ball in play with adroit lever strokes. But most of all I loved that loud distinctive knock, which informed you and the rest of the establishment patrons that you had, in fact, bested the machine and won a game. I removed a dollar from my pocket and slipped it into the machine. Pinball cost a quarter when I had last played. Almost magically, my energy surged as I became the proverbial pinball wizard, deftly knocking the little silver ball back into the bumpers and lights, just like the old days. I felt the warmth of passion glow inside of me as my food grew cold. For the first time in a while, I experienced the simple joy of living, and it felt wonderful.

Often it is those little things that gave us joy that we systematically remove from our life as we resign ourselves to its drudgery. Passion is not all about conquering the world but enjoying its gifts. How many times do we get so caught up in what the poet William Wordsworth refers to as "getting and spending" that we do not take the time to do the things that would give us pleasure? Often, some activity—a hobby, recreation, something that we really like to do—can serve to ignite our passion. It might sound cliché, but passion does involve taking time out to smell the "coffee," as we put it in New Orleans. How easy it is to forget about those simple pleasures that we enjoyed and deliberately deny ourselves. We wait for that perfect day when all our desires are fulfilled and standing in a neat little line in front of us before we embrace the joy of living. The sad fact is that if you always wait for the big things to be happy about, you may be waiting a long time.

I remember once taking a favorite leather briefcase of mine to have its zipper repaired. The owner of the store ran his hands very carefully over the briefcase as he examined the zipper. He then pronounced the briefcase worthy of repair. I had bought it in Ensenada while traveling in Mexico and could never find one that I liked as much. When the owner presented it back to me and observed my reaction to having a favorite briefcase restored, he seemed very content. I realized that he was passionate about his work, even if some might consider it inconsequential. His joy extended beyond the mere twenty bucks he charged me. I wanted to feel the same passion about my work.

The good news is that midlife can often offer you a second chance at passion. It is not uncommon for people to switch careers at midlife and pursue an entirely different line of work. Some go back to school to obtain advanced degrees, so that they can teach. The *Wall Street Journal* ran an article a few years ago about a lawyer becoming a doctor, which I discuss in more detail later. His new undertaking was far from easy and required that he go back to school for his premed courses before even applying to medical school. However, he had the courage to stop a career in midstream and make an about-face. A friend of mine's wife suddenly left a secure corporate position to study nursing while she was in her forties. Although they were financially secure, she still endured the rigors of nursing school and the demanding profession because that had become her midlife calling. On the other hand, people also leave the medical field for other occupations. The truth is that it is never too late to change your occupation.

Ideally, one would have settled on a career that they loved and then stuck to it. But it doesn't always work that way. Many people have more than one career. The late Sonny Bono liked to point out that he had three successful careers. The first was as an entertainer, with his wife, Cher. Their entertainment career actually had several ups and downs. After their recording career sagged, they reinvented themselves with a variety show that started with a modest nightclub act to pay the bills. The "right" person attended one evening and felt that their chemistry would work on television, and it did. Eventually they split up and Sonny went into the restaurant business. Although his restaurant was successful, the cumbersome regulatory process involved in opening the business irritated him. Sonny wanted to fight City Hall and decided to enter politics. He initially was elected mayor of Palm Springs, then in 1994 was elected to the United States Congress. As you know, Sonny Bono died tragically in a skiing accident in 1998, but his remarkable life illustrates how someone with little formal education can become successful in many occupations. Sonny Bono was definitely a passionate as well as successful man. Cher has done very well for herself also, crossing over to acting and winning an Academy Award.

One of the most profound statements about passion that I ever heard was spoken by a woman who is a very courageous survivor of breast cancer. She said that she no longer simply "lived" each day—she "squeezed them dry!" What a wonderful statement by an exceptional woman! That is what passion for living is all about. My grandmother once told me to find something to be happy about every day. Unfortunately, too many of us view life from the opposite angle—that is, we instead look for things to be miserable about.

Healthy vs. Unhealthy Passion

> God grant me the courage to change the things I can change, the serenity to accept those I cannot change and the wisdom to know the difference.
> —Attributed to Adm. Chester W. Nimitz, *The Armed Forces Prayer Book*, motto of Alcoholics Anonymous

It is important to distinguish between healthy and unhealthy passion. Passion is embracing the rush of life and enjoying those things that give us joy. It involves working towards constructive goals for the right reasons.

On the other hand, unhealthy passion—i.e., obsession—can involve an unhealthy preoccupation with someone or something. In many cases, obsession can actually be destructive and even dangerous. Be passionate about your spouse or significant other but not obsessed. Be passionate about your career but not obsessed. Passion and obsession can be easily confused, because many obsessive people seem very successful, at least on the surface. But dig a little deeper and you discover that their lives are completely out of balance. They generally are not happy because they are so consumed with their particular preoccupation, at the expense of the rest of their life.

In reflecting back, I realized that many of my own

achievements were based more upon obsession than passion. As a student, I felt intense pressure to succeed. I wanted to distinguish myself academically from those I considered more affluent. Even in grammar school, I was obsessed with winning one of the plaques awarded to the top three students in each class. In fifth grade, I was intensely competing against someone for third place, the last of the plaques. I became totally obsessed with at least a "show" that year, to borrow horseracing terminology, and eventually did finish third. But although I may have been a bit "smarter" that year, my classmate was far wiser. While I was obsessed with defeating him, he correctly pointed out that a fifth-grade plaque would not make that much difference when we were older. He was right. My passion for succeeding in school was not healthy. It was obsession.

The problem is that obsession robs you of perspective. It is important to keep matters in perspective when you are pursuing your goals, and that is why perspective is an important tune-up step. The obsessed individual is prepared to pay any costs for a particular goal. Perspective helps you temper your passion with some common sense. In a society that promotes instant gratification, it is so easy to lose perspective in the rush to achieve a particular goal. The obsessed individual is prepared to take any shortcut to their perceived "Promised Land."

Consider the many people who become obsessed with losing weight and are willing to do anything to change the scales. This includes taking dangerous medications for quick weight loss (that they were very likely to gain back) as opposed to implementing long-term lifestyle changes of exercise and diet, which are more sustainable and produce healthier results. Diet drugs such as Phen-fen and Redux were reluctantly cleared by the FDA and marketed aggressively by the drug companies. People flocked to the new diet medications without a second thought, but disastrous side effects were discovered, including serious heart conditions.

People who are not obsessed are not necessarily conditioning themselves to fail. Rather, they simply are approaching their desires from a healthier standpoint. They're shooting high but are prepared for whatever happens. They understand that life lessons often arrive through different people and circumstances. They are also aware that the universe some-times has different plans for them than their immediate desires. That is why it is so important to keep perspective even in the midst of aggressively pursuing your most desired goals. As hard as it might be, you sometimes have to stand back, consider your goals in a larger context, and be patient in your quest. Impatience can often turn passion into obsession.

My early political ambitions started with a passion that even-tually degenerated into obsession. I was content in my legal career until my best friend was elected to the legislature. He had run a brilliant campaign, emerging strongly from a crowded field to pull off a stunning political upset. We had campaigned together for other candidates while in college and graduate school and often talked about running for office ourselves. But after he actually got elected, I *had* to get elected also. Although I would have been a capable and hon-est public servant, the prestige of the position motivated me. It was almost as if my life had instantly become incomplete because I wasn't a public official. I resolved to run during the next election cycle, and I *had* to win. However, I encoun-tered problems everywhere I turned. First of all, I lived in a district with a popular incumbent as well as limited opportu-nity for advancement to other offices. So I needed to move into another district. I drove myself crazy trying to find the perfect district and assess vulnerable incumbents or those who were looking to run for other offices. I wanted nothing less than a straight line to an office at the next to election date, and I was forcing the issue.

I later realized that politics is all about timing, and this was simply not a good time. My employer did not want me to run, and a decision to leave them would be very costly. In addi-tion, I would really be pushing it to move into a new district and try to establish myself in time for the next election. However, I lost all perspective as I obsessed and obsessed about the goal.

A few years later, legislative reapportionment created a new seat in my area. The timing was much better in my life for the challenge of a grueling campaign. I campaigned hard for the seat and ended up winning in the first primary against four other challengers. I found out firsthand that God's delays are not necessarily God's denials. When I eventually won, I had more maturity and knowledge to succeed in the position.

Addiction is another form of unhealthy passion. Too many people try to inject passion in their lives with harmful habits. They try to create that missing spark in their lives with such things as an illicit affair, gambling, or substance abuse. The allure of crack cocaine and a gambling addiction cratered the career and family of one of the best trial lawyers I've ever known. This is not to say that all drinking and gambling are bad, just most of it. The key is balance. My grandmother had a tremendous passion for gambling. However, she knew her limits and was able to gamble responsibly on a fixed income. But not everyone can. Some lose their houses and businesses. Unfortunately, addiction is a major problem in our society, and we will talk more about it in the emotional tune-up portion of this book.

Passion Comes from the Core

> Man is only truly great when he acts from the passions.
> —Benjamin Disraeli

Although passion comes from within, it can be stimulated by outside influences. New information, new ideas, new insights, new contacts, new realizations, and new dreams can reinvigorate your life and help you achieve true success. I remember a friend who became quite energized by the movie *Erin Brockovich*. She didn't have a formal education and had always worked in mundane jobs. Once she saw how an uneducated and unsophisticated legal assistant could succeed through determined effort, she became very interested in advancing her own career. Her reaction is called "modeling," which involves imitating the ideas and aspirations of others. There is nothing wrong with modeling the behavior of very successful people. Often, by observing successful people, we can become inspired ourselves. I like to read books or watch programs regarding the biographies of successful people, because I find it energizes my own core.

We can also learn a great deal about passion by observing children. Watch them on the playground, scurrying from swing sets to monkey bars with their eyes all lit up in excitement. They are passionate about their play because no one has yet told them not to be.

Too many of us approach life with trepidation instead of passion. Any tentative flickers of passion can be quickly extinguished the moment we receive any negative feedback from the world. How easy it is to retreat to a comfort zone, where we feel safe but not necessarily complete. Hesitancy can paralyze the choice of a mate, a career change, a financial destination, or any personal aspiration. However, the person who is truly passionate perseveres despite failure and difficulty because the passion lies so deep within them and is part of their being. Despite setbacks, their passion keeps them going.

Many times in my life I felt empty and without passion. It seemed I was always fighting against life's current, and I was quickly tiring. For some reason, I had decided that life would be a struggle, and my beliefs were making this a reality. Of course, if you think that life is a struggle, it will quickly oblige you and could sabotage your efforts. Passion can help you persist during the difficult times and search out the solutions instead of being overwhelmed by the problems.

I learned a good lesson about passion from a client of mine who embodies the epitome of passion. Just a few years ago, he was flat on his back physically, emotionally, and financially. He had just undergone serious neck surgery and wore a neck brace. He and his wife had become divorced after a long marriage that produced three children. The company to which he had given nearly twenty years of excellent service had been sold and the only thanks he received for his hard work was ninety days' severance. He found himself sleeping on a friend's couch.

However, he came roaring back in a few short years. He cashed out his 401(k) plan in order to buy a tugboat. The tug did well and he later leveraged it to purchase half of a struggling marine company. A year later, he bought the other half, leveraging the assets he acquired. Within a few years he had increased the value of his investment by an astounding 5,000 percent and now owns one of the fastest-growing marine companies in the country. Although he became a close friend, I couldn't help but wonder why he was doing so well while I felt so stalled. He appeared to be just a regular guy with no formal education. But his secret to success was his intense passion. I realized just how deep his passion was when he took me fishing.

He was still on his way up at the time and owned a modest fishing boat instead of the sixty-foot yacht he has now. We fished for a while in the marshy area where the Mississippi River meets the Gulf of Mexico. On our way back in, the tide changed and our boat became stuck in the marsh. I am not an experienced fisherman but quickly sensed from his reaction that things were not good. He instructed me to bail everything from the boat in order to gain some buoyancy and free it from the muck. Unfortunately, we remained firmly stuck. Although I didn't think our lives were in any immediate danger, the sun was going down and we were getting increasingly assaulted by mosquitoes. We were facing a long and perhaps very unpleasant ordeal.

My friend suddenly jumped into the waist-deep water and began rocking the boat. I felt obliged to do the same too but was not happy to be in the knee-deep muck. He was pushing and rocking hard. I was doing my best but was distracted by our plight. I kept wondering what the hell I was doing out there in the first place and was angry that he got us in this position. I know that he was a big risk taker. While I admired his risk taking in business, I was less excited when my *own* hide was on the line. He ignored the immobile boat and kept pushing. He instructed me to get back in and help steer, which I was not necessarily unhappy to do. He pushed and pushed. His face grew crimson as he gave a final heave. The boat miraculously eased free and he instructed me to steer it towards the channel. Exhausted, he sank to his knees, his face barely above the surface. For a moment, I thought I might have to abandon the boat and dive in after him. He eventually regained his strength and swam to the boat, and we made it safely back to the dock.

That fishing trip made a deep impression on me. I realized just how immense his heart was as he gave every part of his fiber into pushing the boat free, which initially seemed like an impossible task. I understood why he was so successful, courageously challenging daunting odds with no thought of failure. How could anyone with so much passion fail? I had just witnessed an unforgettable display of passion, and I was awed.

CHAPTER 5

Step 2: Purpose

If one advances confidently in the direction of their dreams and endeavors to lead a life which they have imagined, they will meet with a success unexpected in common hours.

—Henry David Thoreau

(n.) The proper activity of a person or thing; what one intends to do or achieve; goal.

Purpose = Vision

Your passion can be quickly ignited by discovering your purpose. Your purpose is very much related to your vision for your life and the reason that you are here. We have all been endowed with unique skills, and our purpose is to pursue these to the best of our ability. One illustration of purpose appeared in the movie *City Slickers,* which dealt with a group of men coming to grips with midlife issues at a rugged dude ranch. In one scene, Billy Crystal talked with their guide and mentor, played by Jack Palance, about the meaning of life. Palance held up his index finger and informed Crystal that his finger represented "It." When Crystal questioned him, Palance replied that once you figured out what "It" was, your life was set. "It," of course, is your purpose.

Discovering your purpose can be literally life changing. What a thrill it is to match your interests, gifts, and abilities with the unique role that you have carved out in your life. Often in determining your purpose, you have to be totally honest with yourself. Are you happy with what you are doing? Or do you see yourself doing something else? Many self-help books pose the following question about purpose. If there is anything in the world that you would do if you knew that you could not fail, what would it be?

There is no shortage of those searching for their purpose, judging from the enormous success of *The Purpose Driven Life,* which is an excellent book and a must-read for anyone who is searching out their purpose.

Imagine waking up every day excited about the challenges ahead of you, which can happen when you are pursuing your purpose. The problem is that many people do not wake up so eager to face their day. Many feel trapped in careers they might have chosen as teenagers. Now they feel they have no choice but to continue. After all, that's where they started. But would you ask a teenager for career advice? There is no reason to remain in a career you may have chosen years earlier. An important aspect of the midlife tune-up is reevaluating your life and perhaps directing it towards your true purpose. Sometimes, your purpose is right under your nose. In other cases, a bit of reflection and even research are required to ferret it out.

You are the only one who can decide your purpose in life. Often, well-meaning parents, friends, and even spouses can unknowingly detour your personal journey by advising you according to their idea of your purpose. Don't necessarily ignore all outside information, because it is always helpful to consult knowledgeable people. But such opinions need to be integrated with your own decision-making process.

One's purpose is an internal, subjective decision, some-times arrived at more intuitively than intellectually. Sometimes your purpose can be quite specific, such as the choice of being an architect. Other times it is more general, such as starting a business that helps people.

Sometimes constructing your true purpose doesn't involve a total gutting of your career but a simple renovation or even a minor touchup. For example, you might like your occupation but be tired of your industry. Someone who is bored with an accounting position in a large industrial company might become quite fascinated with the entertainment industry. Alternatively, someone might decide they would rather teach accounting but need a doctorate to obtain a tenure-track position. At one point, I felt burnt out as a corporate lawyer and took a battery of career tests administered by an occupational specialist. Imagine my surprise when she concluded that I should—*gasp!*—be a corporate lawyer. I just needed to find a new environment and new challenges. When I accepted an in-house position with a dynamic, growing company, the storm clouds vanished.

Some career changes can be more drastic. I earlier mentioned the *Wall Street Journal* article about an attorney who abandoned his legal career at midlife to become a physician. To make the task even more difficult, the attorney didn't even have the undergraduate prerequisites to get into medical school. He had to start right from the beginning, taking his premed courses at night before even applying to medical school. Then there were four years of medical school and his internship and residency. By all accounts, he was facing a quite daunting and arduous road that seemed ludicrous for anyone in their right mind. But the force that propelled him was a simple mental image of himself in his white coat, making rounds in the hospital. The image was strong and his purpose was undeniable. He had no choice but to follow it and then benefit from the deep sense of satisfaction his decision provided. What strong images do you have of yourself? Many people quite clearly picture the desired images of themselves but are simply afraid to pursue them.

I once watched an interview with a comedian and successful television personality, Jon Stewart. The entertainment industry is perhaps one of the most competitive and difficult areas to succeed in. So many have imagined themselves as entertainment stars but so few actually try. Those who do try struggle for years to get any type of recognition in this fast-paced and unforgiving environment. During the interview, Stewart was asked about the turning point in his career. He stated that it occurred the moment he realized that television was his purpose and that he was totally committing to it. He then put aside all thoughts of failure and distractions and focused wholeheartedly on his career. Despite the enormous obstacles he faced, he stated that he felt quite relieved after this commitment to his purpose. And once he had committed, things finally began to fall into place in his career. Such a moment of truth can often be a liberating as well as intimidating experience, and those who are committed are much more likely to succeed. On the other hand, the road is littered with failures who refused to make such a commitment.

A key benefit of work experience is that it provides an actual reference point of the things that you enjoy doing and, of course, the things you don't. Do you enjoy interacting with people, solving problems, or creating things? The classic best-selling job book entitled *What Color Is Your Parachute?* provides some valuable exercises for determining one's true purpose. By working the exercises, one can determine the type of job they would be interested in. My earlier book, entitled *Break the Curve,* was directed at budding entrepreneurs trying to start a business. I advised that starting a business was hard work, and in order to succeed, one needed to love either the product or the process. Some may be attracted to certain industries or products, such as jewelry, the restaurant industry, or computers. Alternatively, a career can be built around a process, such as selling or analyzing data. A career change could be driven by transferring an existing set of skills to a different industry. On the other hand, you might know your industry very well but are interested in another position. For example, you might be tired of finance in your industry and wish to get into marketing. You'd be amazed at how such an approach can serve to "freshen up" your career.

If you still do not have a clue as to what your purpose should be, explore every avenue of interest to you. Read. Study. Inquire about different activities or careers. And don't give up. There is a purpose out there for you and you just have to find it. As I mentioned earlier, *The Purpose Driven Life* can be an excellent resource in your search.

Commit to Your Purpose

> Why not go out on a limb? Isn't that where the fruit is?
> —Frank Scully

> You will recognize your own path when you come upon it, because you will suddenly have all the energy and imagination you will ever need.
> —Jerry Gillies

Sometimes the problem isn't a lack of purpose but burdening yourself with too many and even conflicting pursuits. Your true purpose can become buried beneath a mound of distractions and activities. Those who spread themselves too thin often end up accomplishing very little. Successful individuals are able to focus on a single purpose, such as building a particular business or starting a new career. This does not mean that they ignore their families or the other important parts of their lives, but they direct most of their attention to *results* for their primary purpose.

Trying to balance too many different activities only seems to diffuse your efforts and your energy. Purpose involves searching for your own uniqueness and then focusing on it. As I well know, it is very easy to sabotage your purpose by cluttering your life with activities.

You will need to decide the overriding purpose in your life, whether it involves real-estate development or sales, for example. If you have more than one dominant purpose, it is much more difficult to succeed. How many people have been successful trying to start three companies at the same time? A few people can balance all of this and pull it off, but it's rare.

Also, you might need to make a living while you are pursuing your purpose. Novelist Patricia Cornwell worked in law enforcement while she wrote the first of her best-selling books. Her "day job" provided not only a means of support but enriched her with knowledge and experience to make her crime novels much more authentic. But she knew all along that her purpose was to be a novelist. And she has been quite successful in her pursuit.

One part of my own tune-up was rediscovering my purpose. In my case, it was not that I didn't have a purpose—I had too many. I was presenting continuing-education seminars around the country, working on a master's degree in accounting systems, lobbying at the state capitol, starting an online learning company, writing educational programs for CPAs, teaching in college, practicing law, planning to enter the political arena as a candidate, as well as writing. I become tired just listing all the activities, let alone doing them. I became quite adept at starting projects but terrible at completing them. I found myself bouncing among an endless array of meetings, seminars, and events. I would go to any lengths to avoid actually sitting down and completing a task. My ridiculous juggling act was my exhausting way of avoiding commitment. Maybe if I did enough projects, one of them might work out well. Of course, none of them did. I realized that I needed to stop juggling and choose.

Obviously, if I was going to get anywhere I needed to radically prune my to-do list. My challenge was to sift through the myriad activities I was burying myself in and choose my purpose. When I was planning my legislative race, I knew that I needed to prioritize my effort if I was to be successful. Several candidates being mentioned were better known and would be better funded than me. I was also not the choice of the political power structure and would be pitted against them and their resources. To make myself more viable against such odds, I planned to clear the decks and spend nearly a year campaigning. At first, no one really took me seriously, thinking I was in over my head. I ignored the skepticism and realized that I needed to start early and focus. And that is exactly what I did, one voter at a time. It paid off on election day, when I received nearly 49 percent of the vote in the first primary against four opponents, finishing twenty points ahead of the political-machine-backed candidate, who later withdrew. I next thought about my legal career, making a decision to become general counsel of a growing marine company so that I could focus on a particular client. Although I had been burned before by going "in house," this opportunity involved a smaller company where I was a member of management. With regards to my writing, I had actually been successful in publishing several business books as well as educational materials. I decided that I would write every day and focus on something that I really wanted to write, which was this book.

I ditched all the rest. What I decided to take on was probably a bit much, but it represented real progress for me.

In choosing your purpose, it is important to focus on the higher-payoff activities and then delegate the rest. During the times when I felt stalled, I was lugging briefcases, knapsacks, and a laptop computer to multiple office suites. But I was getting nothing done. I realized I was not utilizing available administrative and paralegal staff well. I had difficulty starting the more intricate tasks and even greater difficulty completing them. I began delegating as much as I could.

By midlife, you generally have a pretty good idea of what

you're good at and what you're not. Perhaps you've even begun to focus on a specialty that you can perform well. My professional background was as a corporate and tax attorney as well as a CPA. I didn't prepare tax returns but specialized in business planning of closely held entities. Although I wasn't particularly up to date with all the intricacies of personal income taxes, I felt obligated to do my own tax return since, after all, I was a CPA. But individual tax returns require different knowledge from what I had. Tax laws were constantly changing and my return was becoming increasingly complex. Then I found myself at 2:00 A.M. trying to complete my return before the extended August 15 deadline. Just as I thought the end was in sight, my tax software program noted that my return contained a number of discrepancies. That was it. I finally realized how crazy all this was. When I considered how much time I was spending on my return (not to mention the agony), I realized that I'd be much better off using a CPA who specialized in individual tax returns. I applied for another extension and handed my return over to a CPA friend. The extra deductions that he found for me paid for his services a few times over.

Specialize on your purpose, then delegate the rest. Finding the right people to help you can be critical to your success. The key to accomplishing anything meaningful is to focus on your purpose.

Dare to Dream

> Far better it is to dare mighty things, to win glorious triumphs, even though checkered by failure, than to take rank with those poor spirits who neither enjoy much nor suffer much, because they live in the gray twilight that knows not victory nor defeat.
>
> —Theodore Roosevelt

If you set average goals, then you are destined to live an average life. Noted business writer Jim Collins urges his readers to challenge themselves with big, hairy, audacious goals, which he calls *BHAG*. Generally, it is these big goals that can really ignite your passion. That is the unique interplay between passion and purpose, where they can drive each other and produce a combustion of success.

The primary reason why many avoid setting lofty dreams is the fear of failure. Many of the lessons about purpose and self-doubt are not new. As the well-known motivational speaker Tony Robbins notes, "Success leaves clues." Those who succeeded dedicated themselves to a lofty purpose and then focused all their energy on doing their best. They tackled their dreams with optimism and enthusiasm.

If you could do anything in the world and not fail, what would it be? What is something that you want so bad, that you only whisper about it? In the classic book *Journey to the Centre of the Earth,* by Jules Verne, the exploration team is challenged with the following statement: "Descend, bold traveler, into the crater . . . and you will attain the centre of the earth." In setting your purpose, consider yourself a "bold traveler." Be honest with yourself about your purpose. But also be prepared to take some risks. Don't worry at this point how you are going to achieve your purpose—just set it.

Achieving an important purpose is never easy. Most people do not set their purpose high enough to excite them and stir their passion. I keep a plaque on my desk with an important but simple message: *Dream.* Don't be afraid to dream.

The next simple step in the tune-up process is finding your personal power.

CHAPTER 6

Step 3: Power

In confidence and quietness shall be your strength.

—Isa. 30:15

With audacity, one can undertake anything, but not do everything.

—Napoleon Bonaparte

God favors the bold and strong of heart.

—Gen. Alexander A. Vandegrift

(n.) The capacity to exert an influence; a firm belief in one's own powers; the fact or condition of being without doubt.

Developing Your Personal Power

Personal power is the confidence to pursue your purpose. I spoke earlier about how my lack of confidence affected many decisions and actions in my life. I started off my career quite sure of myself, but as life took its inevitable twists and turns, so did my self-assurance. Self-doubt helped perpetuate the downward spiral in my life. But an important turning point occurred when I realized that I had succeeded in the past and could succeed again if I could regain my authority over my life. Self-confidence leads you to act boldly and decisively, to act as if you cannot fail but instead can overcome obstacles and ultimately succeed.

The term "power" can have a bad connotation, conjuring images of power-hungry business moguls or unscrupulous politicians. Personal power involves self-empowerment, enabling yourself to succeed by instilling in yourself a strong belief that you can in fact accomplish your purpose. A common denominator in most successful people is their strong belief in their ability to succeed. Whenever I believed I could do something, I generally could. But whenever I had strong doubts, I usually failed.

People generally rise (and fall) to the level of their beliefs, achieving to the level that they believe they can and that's about it. Our success is a direct function of our beliefs, and that applies to all areas of life. Developing your personal power involves reclaiming your belief in yourself that you can succeed and have a great life. If you feel that you have had a mediocre life up until now, make the decision to have a great life. What are you waiting for? Decide now to empower yourself to improve the important areas of your life.

Another term for personal power is self-mastery—your ability to draw the best from the most unruly person in your life, yourself. It is ironic that others often have more faith in our abilities than we do. If you lack self-confidence, the road to personal power can be quite elusive. We all experience life-changing events, both positive and negative. If you have received considerable negative feedback, which is the case for most of us, it is not always easy to suddenly begin believing in yourself. Sometimes, developing your confidence requires work, much as athletes train and condition themselves for competition.

The first step to unleashing your personal power is to review past accomplishments, as I did. We have all accomplished exceptional and unusual things. What accomplishments are you most proud of? And don't say that you haven't accomplished anything! Think back. Ask close friends or family members. One of my friends was convinced his life was devoid of any noteworth achievement. I pointed out his parenting skills as well as his deep involvement in his children's activities. He was also a great husband and well respected in the community. Yet he had difficulty believing that he had accomplished anything worthwhile. Another friend undertook almost heroic measures in caring for a sick parent. When I pointed out the value of her efforts, she shrugged it off at first. When I persisted, she grudgingly admitted that, although it was difficult, her family was most appreciative. So give yourself credit. Others do. We have all done exceptional things. Review them and be proud. Then resolve to bring your past resourcefulness to the present.

Another way to strengthen your self-confidence is through current accomplishments. Thoreau defined success as the progressive accomplishment of worthwhile goals. There is much wisdom in this statement, which breaks down success into a series of goals. Accomplishing one goal can help you attain the next, more difficult one. And don't forget to celebrate any incremental success. Often, we become so focused on the desired outcome, we forget to congratulate ourselves for the important steps leading to our purpose. New England Patriots coach Bill Belichick, who has won three Super Bowls, stated that it wasn't the actual Super Bowl he most enjoyed so much as working on the day-to-day football fundamentals. He was able to string these small daily victories into world championships.

In their rush to get ahead, people often forget that success consists of gradual steps. As you begin meeting your interim goals, you become more confident. Budding politicians don't run for governor—they run for local offices and gradually work their way up. The same is true with entrepreneurs at every level. They usually have accumulated several small successes as part of their desired outcome.

Planning, the next simple step in the tune-up process, involves dividing your ultimate goal into smaller pieces to be pursued and accomplished. This incremental approach helps you enjoy each level of success. Such a systematic and stratified approach makes your ultimate goal or purpose that much easier to obtain, and you become empowered along the way. When I started writing again, the thought of completing an 80,000-100,000-word manuscript felt quite overwhelming, particularly writing on a part-time basis. But this seemingly impossible task was made quite possible when a speaker at a writer's conference pointed out that composing one page a day could produce a completed book in a year. Breaking a larger goal into its component pieces makes it more achievable and therefore helps to reduce your fear and uncertainty.

Note your accomplishments every step of the way, as this can provide you with the confidence to persist. While running for office, I realized that every person who agreed to vote for me—or better yet, put up a lawn sign or made a contribution— brought me one step closer to my goal of winning the election.

I always lugged around lawn signs so that I could put them up as soon as someone agreed. This helped provide the confidence I needed to go up against the political machine.

Success in one area of your life can bring success in another. For example, the better I was able to stick to my physical-exercise regimen, the better I felt about myself and the more successful I was in my career. As I enjoyed small successes, pursued balance, and developed a strong belief in myself, my life soon began to purr along in a synergistic fashion. I found that once I empowered myself, the other parts of my life began to work together. As I gained confidence, I started making better decisions. Gone were those feelings of being stuck in life as I continually agonized over decisions. When I didn't trust my decision-making ability, I ended up making poor decisions. I found that I was rushing them, not taking the time to outline all of the ramifications. When my confidence returned, I started making better decisions.

In fact, decision making can help increase your confidence. It can be easy to become immobilized over the thought of failure and the results of making a bad decision. Confident people are decisive and able to make quick decisions. This is not to say that they are always right, because no one is going to make perfect decisions. But your decision commits you to a course of action. During one of my spiritual retreats, I confided to a retreat master that I had great difficulty making a decision. The wise priest, who used to chair the psychology department at Loyola University in New Orleans, told me that the only way to overcome the fear of making decisions was to make decisions. During the times when I felt my lowest, I couldn't even decide what to eat that day. I had totally abdicated all of my decision-making power. I was afraid to decide anything for fear of making a mistake. A serious relationship stayed in a limbo state far too long because I couldn't figure out what to do. Eventually, the decision about the relationship was made for me. Personal power is about reclaiming your belief in yourself. Making decisions is a step in the belief process.

Some people are born with great power and confidence, but for others it has to be developed. I sometimes watch the VH-1 television program entitled "Behind the Music," which chronicles the lives of rock stars. The pattern is often quite predictable. For the young artist, there is struggle and obscurity and then a burst of fame, which often comes at a steep price. Many of the stars are simply too immature to handle the prominence and wealth suddenly thrust upon them. Their system overloads and they cope with substance abuse. Their career and sometimes their lives hit the proverbial dead-end.

It is rare to find an entertainer who can climb to the top and stay there. And one such performer, whether you like her or not, is Madonna. She is also a great illustration of just how far personal power can take a career. Even if you don't approve of her lifestyle or image, you cannot deny the enormous impact she has had on popular culture and her lofty status as an entertainer.

While I was watching a VH-1 special on Madonna, I realized that the seeds of her success were sown while she was very young, primarily due to her intense confidence and will. The most revealing thing about her as a person was her first appearance on "American Bandstand" at the age of twenty-one. Dick Clark thrust a microphone in her face and asked, "What do you want to do?" Now, what do you think she said? To have a hit record? At that time she didn't have any hits and was still basically an unknown. Was it to have a successful recording career? She had just signed with her label and was far from a success.

No, Madonna's answer was: "I want to rule the world."

This might seem a quite ambitious thing for an unknown twenty-one-year-old to say. But guess what? In Madonna's own way, she did go on to rule the world. She certainly has ruled the entertainment world. She has had numerous hits and blazed her own trail in popular culture. The interesting thing is that if you dissect Madonna as an entertainer, you can find many reasons why she should not have done as well as she did. Let's start with her voice. Many singers in the entertainment world have better ones. Consider her appearance. Although Madonna is obviously a pretty woman who is aging well, there are certainly other singers out there who are much more attractive. By entertainment standards, she is far from drop-dead gorgeous.

More than anything else, her success was driven by her will and her confidence—her personal power. She developed her own unique style and she never had any doubt that she was going to succeed. She left her home and went to New York in search of fame and fortune. She did what she had to do to survive, and that included eating out of trashcans, dating the right people, or going to the right nightclubs to meet certain record producers. Despite the obstacles she faced, she maintained tremendous belief in herself. This personal power separated her from scores of emerging performers. Many new singers tried to imitate Madonna's style. They may have had one or two hits, but their careers soon fizzled. I remember a singer named Taylor Dayne who was described in the late 1980s as "the new Madonna." However, the last time I saw her in concert, it was a small venue and there were only a few dozen people there. I actually felt bad for her. She's a beautiful and sexy woman with a good voice. So why did her career tank while Madonna's continues to soar? Much of it stems from Madonna's belief in herself and the sheer force of her will.

Other singers, such as Shania Twain, also had to overcome personal and career difficulties in order to succeed. In many cases, their undying confidence separated them from those who anonymously faded away. The tastes of fickle consumers can literally change overnight. Those entertainers who last possess powerful self-assurance as well as considerable talent. I recently attended a concert by Neil Sedaka in Las Vegas. His peak was a little before my time, but I understand that he was quite a hit in the late 1950s and the early 1960s and his innocent, lighthearted rock music sold 10 million albums. However, in 1964, a British rock group called the Beatles played on "The Ed Sullivan Show." Consumers swarmed to this new brand of rock and roll, and Sedaka vanished for a decade. But Sedaka kept plugging away, doing what he did best, and by the mid-1980s had another best-selling album, appropriately titled *Sedaka's Back*. No one knows the peaks and valleys that can tax one's confidence better than entertainers.

But the key ingredient in all cases is to believe in yourself—to empower yourself.

Overcoming Your Fears

No pain, no palm; no thorn, no throne; no gall, no glory; no cross, no crown.

—William Penn, *No Cross, No Crown*

That which does not kill me makes me stronger.
—Friedrich Wilhelm Nietzsche, *Twilight of the Idols*

To be, or not to be: that is the question:
Whether 't is nobler in the mind to suffer
The slings and arrows of outrageous fortune,
Or to take arms against a sea of troubles,
And by opposing end them?

— Shakespeare

Summoning up and maintaining your confidence is not always easy. Just when you're feeling good, along comes a setback, negative thought, or stab of apprehension to trip up your dreams. Whenever you think about a desired goal or purpose and then decide to pass on it, fear is most likely the culprit. Fear often separates deserving people from their goals. You might be attracted to someone but be afraid to ask them out for fear of being rejected. You might want to try a new career but are afraid to leave your job. Fear comes in many forms: fear of failure, fear of success, and fear of the unknown.

Fear is universal; everyone experiences it at some time in their lives. Even the most seasoned performers report that they still get butterflies before they go on stage. Even the most confident business executives worry that their decisions might not be correct. Often, those who appear the most self-assured are battling significant fear.

The key is to "feel the fear and do it anyway," to borrow the title of a best-selling book by Susan Jeffers. Her research reveals that everyone has fear. But the successful ones are those who have learned to work through their fears. They feel the fear and do it anyway. Fear can definitely immobilize you, if you let it. And it will not simply vanish on its own. Personal power involves the ability to push through your fears.

But this is obviously easier said than done, particularly when the fear is real and gripping. Consider a method to address it. Initially, realize that everyone has fear and that you are not alone in your anxiety. Don't try to avoid or deny your fear— rather, examine it directly. Understand and analyze your fear, and ultimately turn it to your advantage.

So actually, what are you afraid of? Often it can be the

discomfort of venturing outside of our comfort zone or, more specifically, the fear of failure or rejection. We tend to magnify our fear by exaggerating potential negative consequences. Rather than rationally evaluate the risk, we fixate on any possible catastrophic outcome, no matter how remote. Your fear can consume you if you let it. Instead, step back and analyze it. What *really* are you really afraid of? What *really* is the worst thing that can possibly happen? Remember that 90 percent of the outcomes that we fear never happen. Reflect back on your own life and you'll recognize the truth in this statement. How many things did you worry about that never came to pass? Mark Twain once observed, "I've had many terrible experiences in my life, some of which actually happened."

Resolve to *realistically* prepare yourself for the worst. Before attempting anything, ask yourself what is the worst that can actually happen. Can you handle that? This is an important step in reducing the size of your fear. For example, many experience fear when calling on a new business prospect. I certainly do. But ask yourself, what is the worst that can happen? Getting verbally rebuked or being hung up on. That's it. A hangup won't ruin you financially or professionally, and you shouldn't even allow it to ruin your day. If you can handle this fear of rejection, then pick up the phone and make that call.

Suppose you want to run for office. What is the worst that can happen? Of course, you can lose. This is the question I had to face when I ran. I decided that I could handle the loss, emotionally and financially. I budgeted a certain amount to run, which would not ruin me financially, set aside the time, and then took my shot.

Suppose you want to start a business. What is the worst that can happen? The business can fail. If you are putting all of your assets on the line, this could be a considerable risk. But even if you lost it all, do you have the ability to earn it back?

Consider perhaps starting a business as a sideline. What is the worst that can happen? You might lose your initial investment, but not your home. I once counseled a young woman who wanted to start a retail chocolate business, beginning with a cart in a shopping mall. I knew that her husband did well financially and that her initial costs were less than ten thousand dollars. However, she was totally immobilized by the fear of failure, actually to the point of tears in my office. I kept trying to point out that her venture was a reasonable risk that would have little effect on her financial condition. But she remained fixated on the negative. She blew her downside risk totally out of proportion and she never did start her business.

On the other side of the spectrum, I've had clients who were so desperate to start a business they refused even to consider the risks. During the early days of the Internet, I had a client who was ready to risk his entire worth to launch an online learning company. I was also fascinated by the area and had recently attended a major online learning trade show, where I had spoken with many industry leaders. I advised my client that he either needed to raise more money or focus his plan—that to risk his life savings to compete against these giants was foolhardy.

A happy medium is the client I spoke about earlier who invested his life savings in a marine vessel. However, he had spent his whole career in the marine industry, knew the vessel was a bargain, and already had customers lined up for it. He realized a good opportunity when he saw it and was well prepared to take his risk. Of course, he could lose his investment in the vessel, but he felt that his downside risk was reasonable under the circumstances. This is where power and planning interrelate. Careful planning empowers you to take risks. Taking risks without proper planning is foolhardy. I told my client who was desperate to put his life savings into a long-shot online learning venture to go gamble in Las Vegas. At least he'd have a good time.

A physician friend of mine served as a pilot in the Vietnam War. His greatest fear was being captured by a sadistic enemy. This not only makes our own fears pale by comparison but also provided him with a way of coping with the tremendous stress of combat. Once he decided he could handle his greatest fear, the rest seemed easy.

So whenever you feel fear tugging at your stomach, ask yourself what is the worst that can happen. Can you handle that? We all have different risk profiles, and my friend in the marine industry is much more of a risk taker than I am. The key is to take risks that are reasonable in light of your particular circumstances. Once you have corralled that initial fear, you are able to make better judgments about acceptable versus unacceptable risks. There is nothing wrong in turning down an unacceptable risk. Professional investment companies evaluate risk and return of investments all the time, and they too turn down unacceptable risks. But don't let fear of loss cloud your judgment as you make your assessments.

Excessive fear often results from negative thought patterns. If we have a tendency to assume the worst, then our lives could turn into a self-fulfilling prophecy. I've had to struggle with negative thinking most of my life. Even when things were relatively good, I could usually find something wrong. And when life dealt me an inevitable setback, I often reacted disproportionately. Looking back, I realized that most of the worries that consumed me never actually happened. I received an excellent lesson in positive thinking from a young woman who is an inspiration to me. Although she has had several health problems, she remains one of the happiest people I know. Due to a digestive problem, she had to use a portable feeding tube for a number of years. Despite her health issues, she busied herself with raising her family and pursuing her career. Then she was diagnosed with brain cancer. Her spirits remained strong even when she underwent difficult sessions of chemotherapy. My problems at the time seemed to pale by comparison and I actually felt ashamed by some of my negative thinking. Although she went into remission for a while, the cancer returned. I saw her after she and her family returned from a trip to the beach. She told me about an interesting occurrence when she and her daughter were sitting on the beach. A thunderstorm was forming in the Gulf of Mexico, and they happened to be sitting on the beach right at the border of the storm. Their view of the ocean presented stark contrasts. On the left side was the ominous darkness of the approaching storm, but to the right was the dazzling beauty of the summer day. As the storm rolled in towards shore, she wasn't sure whether they were going to have to flee indoors or would be left unscathed by the storm and permitted to remain on the beach. Her daughter was playing beside her on the beach. The little girl saw the approaching storm and became alarmed. "What are we going to do, Mommy?" she asked with a tinge of fear in her voice.

Her mother glanced at the blackness and turbulence on the left and then to the bright blue sky to the right and replied, "Look to the right."

She told me that whenever she has bad times, she resolves to "look to the right." So whenever you find yourself consumed by negative thinking and fear, resolve to "look to the right." If this woman can, you certainly should be able to. Part of overcoming fear involves developing a positive attitude or perspective on life. We will discuss perspective in a later chapter.

Negative thinking, which is tied directly to fear, can often be manifested by negative self-talk. This can prove demoralizing and debilitating. If you're wondering what self-talk is, it is that little voice inside your head that can chatter incessantly. Part of overcoming your fear involves managing the negative self-talk that can create or reinforce it. Although you might not be able to control all of your external circumstances, you can, with some effort, restrain that voice inside your head, particularly during times of agitation and stress. One of the benefits of evaluating your fears is to gain a handle on your thoughts and self-talk. Calm your inner voice down and you will calm yourself down.

Proper planning, which we address in the next chapter, can also help eliminate much of the risk of failure and hence reduce the fear of it. Research by the Small Business Administration indicates that approximately four in five business startups fail. However, 90 percent of these business failures can be traced to poor management. But in my experience as an adviser and mentor to numerous startups, new businesses that plan carefully, execute confidently, and learn quickly from their mistakes have at least an even chance of success.

Planning can also greatly enhance personal power. After you've prepared yourself for the worst, the next step is to prepare to succeed. For example, if you are afraid to speak in public, give practice speeches. Such preparation can provide you with the necessary confidence to do it for real.

I recognized the power of planning when I entered some athletic events later in life. To say I was never much of an athlete is somewhat of an understatement. I was very awkward as a teenager and generally the last one chosen for teams on the playground—not the second to last or third to last but last. In some sense, this lack of physical ability always nagged at me. It led me to set some physical goals later in life.

My first goal in my thirties was to run a marathon, which if you don't know is 26.2 miles. Although I was never a fast runner, I did have endurance. I actually enjoyed running and was doing it regularly, 6 miles at a time. However, to increase from 6 to 26 miles is quite a stretch. I talked with others who had run marathons and inquired about their training schedules. I eventually used a schedule that would vary the length of the run each day and gradually increase the weekly long run until it reached 20 miles. Each week I trained and added a few more miles to my long run, first 10 miles, then 13 miles, and then 15 miles. I gained confidence that I could make it to 26.2 miles. Besides the training, I also needed to learn the tricks of the trade, like putting lubricants on your thighs and protecting sensitive areas of your body from the chafing of sweat-drenched clothes. It is also important to keep your body hydrated and consume vitamin supplements along the way, which prevents you from hitting the dreaded "wall." This is where your body has burned off all energy sources, and it leads to muscular failure that can stop you in your tracks. As it turned out, I did finish the marathon. It took me four hours and twenty-eight minutes. A friend congratulated me as I crossed the finish line, saying I had accomplished something that very few people did. That's not bad for a clumsy kid who was always picked last. I empowered myself through careful training.

In my forties, I set a new athletic goal of triathlons, which combine running, swimming, and biking. The sprint triathlons I trained for involve a 1,000-yard swim, a twenty-mile bike ride, and a three-mile run. While the individual events themselves are not overwhelming, the combination of the three can be a bit daunting. Most people who enter triathlons are pretty good in one or two events but have to train hard for the other. I found the swim to be my biggest challenge. I hadn't swum in years and the event involved swimming in open water. The problem with an open-water swim is that you cannot easily stop and rest if you become tired. I received advice from a swim coach who helped me refine my technique. I quickly fell in love with swimming, particularly after a hot, rough day. However, I realized that there is a key distinction between a swim in a nice, clear pool with the lines at the bottom and a swim in the open water of a dark lake.

The best advice I received was to practice open-water swims *before* the event. I also was told to buy good equipment, which included large goggles that provided peripheral vision and a wetsuit that helped make me more buoyant. Armed with the right advice, equipment, and practice, I felt empowered. I did make the mistake of scheduling a party at my home right after the event, so everyone would know how I had done— or whether I had been done in.

On the day of the triathlon, I was quite nervous. I saw some people from the gym who came to watch the race. They were better athletes than me and stared at me incredulously as I descended into the cold lake before the starting gun. They weren't participating in the event, so what was I doing out there? The current was a little rough. I tried to look confident but was scared to death. I surveyed the markers as I stood nervously in the waist-deep, cold water. They seemed so far away. Most of the course was in ten feet of water. There were boats around to fish out people who got into trouble. How had I gotten myself into this? Then I reminded myself that the swim was 1,000 yards. That is twenty laps. I was up to sixty laps in my practice sessions. Twenty laps was not that big of a deal. My wetsuit provided some extra buoyancy, and I remembered the advice to float on my back if I got into trouble. The starting pistol sounded. I gasped as I plunged into the cold water and for a minute froze up as I struggled to catch my breath. Then I began taking strokes one at a time and fell into my rhythm. Due to the current, I adjusted my breathing to every second stroke, turning my mouth towards the shore. I passed the first marker and turned towards the second. I felt my confidence surge. I was swimming easily and before I knew it had reached the shore. Although I had a twenty-mile bike ride and three-mile run ahead of me, I was elated. I had faced an extreme fear and had prevailed. I had empowered myself through preparation, and when the big day came I was ready. Predictably, the boats around me had fished out those who were not as well prepared and who got into trouble. But I was ready and the swim was a breeze.

I once helped coach a client to sever a business relationship. He was expanding rapidly and wanted to buy out a minority partner but was unable to approach him. I pointed

out that the longer he waited, the more expensive the acqui-
sition would be. My client wanted to make the move but was
unable to take that final step. I knew that he was not good
at difficult conversations, so I helped prepare him. I suggested that he play the role of his associate while I played
him. We rehearsed his responses a few times. The session
helped him to finally approach his associate and negotiate a
buyout. Since that time, his business has increased substantially in value.

If you have a major presentation or even a confrontation
coming up, empower yourself by rehearsing the situation.
You'd be amazed how this can make your confidence soar
and, of course, reduce your fear.

Preparation is the key. Don't be caught flatfooted by someone you are not ready to deal with. It is never a good idea to
make a decision while you are off balance because you are
then acting from weakness instead of strength. Instead, take
the time to regain your footing and steady yourself. Many
salespeople try to trick you into making a decision when you
are off balance. They might insist that the offer is only good
for this immediate time. That is an old negotiation strategy
that nudges you into a decision you might not want to make.

A common situation we all dread is buying a car.
Although some dealers have become more professional,
the showroom can still test your confidence and personal
power. Preparation is the key to getting a good deal on a
car. It used to be that the starting point for negotiating a
car purchase was the "sticker price." The salesperson
would invariably base their negotiation on the sticker
price, which often included several thousand dollars in
profit. Today there is readily available information about
the car's cost, which enables customers to negotiate from
the cost up instead of from the sticker down. Such cost
information as well as comparative shopping can help you
make an informed decision that you are confident about. I
shopped very diligently for my last car. I found an excellently
maintained one with minimal mileage at a price considerably
below the new model. I had carefully studied the pricing
structure for the model and was able to dicker a bit with
the dealer. When I received the dealer's final offer, I knew
for sure that it was an excellent deal and gladly acted to

consummate the purchase. I had no buyer's remorse (for once) because I was prepared.

In the course of my work, I often negotiate tax settlements with the IRS as well as negotiate with other businesses on behalf of clients. I never speak to opposing counsel or the government unless I am ready with all the facts. Otherwise, I am not dealing from a position of strength but rather a position of weakness. When you deal from a position of weakness, you are more fearful and prone to make mistakes. Take the time to prepare so that you can increase your personal power.

CHAPTER 7

Step 4: Planning

If you aim at nothing, you will surely hit it.
—Lt. Gen. Robert H. Forman

(v.) To form a strategy for; to work out and arrange the parts of.

The next simple step in the tune-up process is planning. Although you may be empowered to achieve a purpose that you are passionate about, you can easily squander your good intentions and diligent efforts without proper planning. Proper planning is the basis of personal effectiveness.

Today's hectic world constantly challenges us with time demands. No matter who we are, we have only twenty-four hours in a day and we often find ourselves at war with time, trying to satisfy the crushing demands of our jobs and families. We scurry about to get things done as quickly and efficiently as possible. But *efficiency* is not always the answer. Instead, be *effective* in handling your personal and business matters. Efficiency can be thought of as doing things right, while effectiveness is doing the *right* things. For example, it does little good to do things efficiently that do not need to be done at all. Effectiveness involves making the right choices.

The principle of effectiveness and planning is best explained by noted author and economist Peter Drucker, who is widely regarded as the father of modern management. His book on the subject is aptly titled *The Effective Executive*. Although written in the 1960s, the book is timeless in its wisdom and practical advice on time management and planning.

The bad news, according to Drucker and others who have researched this area, is that most people are not nearly as effective as they can be. However, the good news is that effectiveness can be learned, and the major key to effectiveness is proper time management. Time is the one true scarce resource. We all are given the same amount of time. We cannot produce any more of it, and once it is spent, we can't get it back.

Planning for Effectiveness

> Who begins too much accomplishes little.
> —German proverb

Proper time management or planning for effectiveness can be broken down into a series of steps.

Prioritize. The first component in planning for effectiveness is establishing your priorities. Determine those goals that are centered around your purpose and most important to you. In the next part of this book, we will discuss establishing your purpose in the important areas of your life, which include career, financial, relationships, and spiritual. Once you have established your purpose or goals in each of the important areas of your life, isolate those activities that contribute most to your purpose and then prioritize those activities. Since it is impossible to accomplish everything, focus on those activities that provide the most benefit and move you closer to your purpose.

As I well know, it is often very easy to become distracted from your priorities. We clutter our lives with an array of activities and before long we can become stretched quite thin. Often, lost in the confusion, are the higher-payoff activities that bring us closer to our desired purpose. That is why it is so important to establish your priorities. Focus on your priorities and don't become distracted by collateral activities. We are always tempted to answer phone calls, play on the Internet, read junk mail, or do everything except those activities that are most important to us. Personal effectiveness involves the discipline to focus on your priorities. Effectiveness is not "knocking out" the smaller items before tackling the larger, more important tasks; it is handling the important tasks *first*.

The importance of prioritizing is illustrated by the often-cited Pareto principle, which states that we derive 80 percent of our results from 20 percent of our activities. This principle was advanced by Vilfredo Pareto, a nineteenth-century

Italian economist who formulated it while measuring patterns of wealth and income in England. He found that the majority of the wealth was owned by a small percentage of the people and there was a direct mathematical correlation, namely 20 percent of the population owned 80 percent of the wealth. Pareto analyzed even further and discovered that 80 percent of the wealth of this top 20 percent was itself controlled by 20 percent of this top rung. He also found this 80/20 pattern practically everywhere that he researched. He discovered that 20 percent of the customers produced 80 percent of the sales, 20 percent of the sales produced 80 percent of profit, and so on.

The Pareto principle is one of the most important rules in planning today. Since time demands can be so overwhelming, it is critical to concentrate on higher-payoff activities. Since you cannot possibly accomplish all that you want to, prioritize and plan activities that focus on that magic 20 percent that produces 80 percent of the results.

Log Your Time. Management consultants have recommended logging your time for at least a week to determine exactly how you spend your time. This exercise can be quite revealing. People are often shocked to find that they spend the *most* time on the *least* productive activities. For example, corporate executives are often surprised to discover how little of their time is actually spent on important senior management activities, such as strategic planning for the organization. A time log can help you redirect your activities or even delegate or eliminate them.

Although it might seem tedious, try logging your time for one week to determine exactly how you're spending your time, while monitoring your progress towards your priorities. Are you focusing on that important 20 percent, or are you allowing yourself to be distracted by other, less valuable uses of your time?

Schedule Blocks of Time. Notice that I said *blocks* of time. The point is that the effective individual needs to have disposable time available in fairly large chunks. This is also known as consolidating your time. Despite all the technological advances today, important tasks still require adequate time. How often do we rush through something and make some costly mistake that requires even more time to resolve?

Schedule adequate time to complete your priorities. Considerable time can be wasted by constantly stopping and starting an activity. Block out the time and finish the important activities that you schedule.

Scheduling such blocks of time is not always easy and requires some determination and even cooperation in holding your calls and visitors. Sometimes it is easier to schedule such uninterrupted periods at home. And, of course, the 80/20 principle would be used to determine those critical activities for which uninterrupted planning time is necessary.

Effectiveness requires the planning out of important activities in advance. Plan your work and then work your plan. Establish the desired direction for your career and your life and then follow through on your plans. All of the various goals that you might list in the important areas of your life can be translated into a series of activities. Then schedule the activities. Appendix A provides a guide for properly scheduling and prioritizing your life goals.

An Orderly Life

> Our life is frittered away by detail. . . . Simplify, simplify.
> —Henry David Thoreau, *Walden*

Another important part of planning is putting your life in order. The first step is to get rid of the clutter. It is very easy for our workspaces and homes to become cluttered. Such clutter only serves to weigh us down and prevent us from working on the important things in our lives. Often, I would spend more time looking for things, getting ready to get started, than actually finishing anything. Many projects that appeared daunting initially were actually quite achievable when I was able to break them into steps and then began working on each of the steps. I found that a clean and organized workspace better enabled me to dive into projects than a cluttered one. When things became too messy, I often felt helpless.

Removing the clutter requires the commitment of blocks of time that we talked about earlier. You can't do it a little at a time. The two areas to prioritize are your home and workspace, including your home office. Set aside a block of time to get organized. Many products are available to help you. I still favor expandable and manila folders that contain typed file labels. These labels give the folders a much more important appearance and make you more serious about remaining organized.

You can break up your personal filing into bank accounts, investments, medical, insurance, tax information, and others. It is also possible to rid yourself of paper altogether by scanning and storing information in a digital format. More people are using check-balancing software and paying their bills online. We are gradually moving away from a paper society. The only papers you retain should be the important ones. Many of us allow papers to accumulate for no particular reason, which only bogs us down. Resolve to keep the papers that are most important and discard the rest. Important papers would include originals of certain documents such as insurance policies, warranties, etc. Get rid of everything else. This not only applies to paper but also to clothes and other articles in your life.

There is nothing more distracting from the pursuit of your goals than a messy office or home. If you do have a cluttered lifestyle, one of your highest priorities should be to rid yourself of the clutter. Attack your home room by room. Don't underestimate the time that it will take you. However, the reward is very much worth it. Think of how good you will feel when you rid yourself of all of the accumulated junk that weighs you down.

Incremental Goal Setting

> The person who makes a success of living is the one who sees his goal steadily and aims for it unswervingly. That is dedication.
>
> —Cecil B. De Mille

Since goal setting is so important, it merits some further discussion. There are proven techniques for setting and achieving goals. To begin with, goals need to be:

- Written. Anything that is not in writing is just a wish. Committing your goal to paper is a major step towards its accomplishment.
- Specific. Details are the foundation of goal setting. The

more specific you are in establishing your goals, the more likely you will accomplish them. For example, the goal that you want start exercising to lose weight is not nearly specific enough. Determine how many pounds you want to lose, and commit to a specific exercise program.

- Measurable. The more you can measure your goal, the easier it is to track your progress. It is hard to determine if you have achieved a goal if it cannot be measured. Commercial weight-loss plans, for example, all require daily weigh-ins to track your progress.
- Achievable. Goals need to be realistic. Achievable goals are those that are just out of reach but not out of sight.

Another benefit of such planning is that incremental improvements can add up dramatically. It is so easy to become discouraged in your quest for your dreams, thinking you will never achieve them. Remember, though, that our lives are not always a steady, upward progression. Sometimes our path can be a bit jagged as we have to travel from peak to peak. Although you may feel a bit stalled at the time, concentrate on completing important activities a little better each day. Such incremental improvements can add up to measurable progress in our lives and eventually yield a dramatic result. For instance, even if you are aiming to lose twenty pounds, losing ten pounds of fat and adding muscle can tremendously improve your appearance in the meantime, as well as your outlook. Incremental improvements in each of the important areas of your life create a synergy of self-improvement and keep your life in balance.

Goal setting yields the best results when you plan on a daily basis. In an age of PCs, Palm Pilots, BlackBerries, Outlook, and other personal information managers, there is no excuse for not taking time to plan. Planning involves the following steps.

1. Decide on the major goals or purposes in your life in each of the important areas:
   a. Emotional
   b. Financial
   c. Career
   d. Relationship

    e. Physical

    f. Mental

    g. Spiritual

  2. Prioritize your goals.

  3. Break down each goal into activities.

  4. Schedule the activities.

Review your goals on a weekly basis and plan your week in advance. While the bulk of your schedule will include career or work projects, don't neglect the other aspects of your life, such as exercising, meeting with a financial planner, or watching an educational program on television. Plan recreational activities, such as movies or dates with your spouse or significant other during the middle of the week. This can refresh you and keep you going.

Also, don't use a planning system that is too cumbersome. I once tried to use a complicated color-coded life-planning system. I ended up more disorganized than before and finally abandoned it. The most advanced organizing system won't benefit you if you don't use it. For many, simply jotting a to-do list for the upcoming day works just fine. Alternatively, you might find a planning system or software that suits you.

Once a week, review your major goals and then plan the activities for the next week. This simple system is often underutilized. Regular planning increased my own effectiveness and it can increase yours also. Without a plan, I found myself too easily distracted by whatever arose. Planning helps you to distinguish between the urgent (activities demanding immediate attention) and the important (high-payoff activities that will help you accomplish your purpose). Often, things that appear urgent, such as unimportant phone calls that get buzzed through or a stack of mail that is placed on your desk, are really not important. But they tend to pull at you like a powerful magnet. Before you know it, you have wasted a lot of time and not gotten around to the important things. Effectiveness involves deflecting the urgent but unimportant activities and returning to your priorities.

Remember, although you may not be able to achieve *everything* you want, you can achieve practically *anything* you want if you plan effectively.

CHAPTER 8

Step 5: Perspective

Enjoy your own life without comparing it with that of another.

—Marquis De Condorcet

There is nothing either good or bad, but thinking makes it so.

—Shakespeare

(n.) A frame of mind affecting one's thoughts or behavior.

Perspective = Attitude

As I mentioned earlier, just about every self-help book I ever read extols the virtues of a positive attitude. But there is a good reason for this. Your attitude is your filter to the outside world, through which interactions, ideas, and experiences are interpreted. Simply put, those with a positive attitude tend to see the good in situations, while those with a negative attitude focus on the bad. Remember the earlier advice about "look to the right." All other things being equal, those who are positive and look for the good in all situations are generally much more successful than those with a negative attitude. A positive attitude or perspective can tremendously boost your quality of life, since your attitude is the foundation of your actions, thoughts, and feelings.

This interplay between positive and negative can be illustrated in the Chinese symbol of the yin and the yang:

99

In the symbol, the flip side of challenge is opportunity. It is far more constructive to approach challenges or setbacks as opportunities instead of as tragedies. It is much better to pick up the broken pieces and move on than to continue to mope about your bad fortune. It is your attitude or perspective that governs your world view and whether you interpret events positively or negatively. A positive attitude can serve as our impenetrable fortress against any arrows that life shoots at us.

The American version of the yin and the yang is the bottle that is either half-full or half-empty. It is far easier to dwell on the things we don't have than to give thanks for our blessings. It is easy to become preoccupied with scarcity instead of grateful for prosperity, spending much of our lives steeped in regret. People regret their spouses, their careers, decisions they made, decisions they didn't make, risks they took, and risks they didn't take. They feel they have somehow missed out on what their life was supposed to be. The good news is that people are living longer and more productive lives and have the opportunity to learn from their experiences and positively redirect their lives. Resolve to analyze your life experience, learn from it, put it behind you, and move forward.

Too many of us dwell on the past, ignore the present, and fear the future.It is much more productive to learn from the past, enjoy the present, and plan for the future. Your previous life experience, no matter how painful or costly, can prove to be a valuable learning tool to help you plan for the future.

Such life experience provides clearer insight into boom and bust cycles, because you've lived through them. I once listened to an experienced business owner mentor a younger entrepreneur about expanding too rapidly during a boom period in their particular industry. He cautioned about becoming overleveraged because he remembered the "bad times" and that all business was cyclical. Chances are that by midlife you're much wiser and in a position to capitalize on that, since experience is often the best teacher. But don't get mired in your mistakes and problems from the past. We all have had our occasional ruts. Failure and mistakes can be great teachers, if you view them from the proper perspective. For example, you may have failed in a certain career or undertaking. But that just makes you wiser the next time. Just because things in your life didn't work out earlier doesn't necessarily mean they can't work out now.

I know firsthand how hard it can be to keep morale up during those difficult times when you feel trapped in a dead-end career, a failing relationship, or worse. Some mornings, I could barely get out of bed. Although such times can be quite testing, a positive attitude combined with other steps of the tune-up process, such as planning and power, can be your most effective means of escape. I have always turned to God during my most difficult times, and He has never denied me. This is not to say that all my problems were immediately solved, but I was filled His grace and faith and, with them, the courage, strength, and hope to face another day. I discuss the powerful benefits of a God-centered life in the spiritual tune-up chapter.

Two self-help classics provide penetrating insights into the importance of attitude. *The Road Less Traveled,* by M. Scott Peck, begins with the sobering but accurate sentence, "Life is hard." Because they grew up during prosperous times, many baby boomers have instead been conditioned to believe that "life is good and it's supposed to get better." They never lived through the challenges and scarcity of the Great Depression or the threat to our freedom of World War II. Sometimes it is simply too easy to become rattled by life's inevitable hardships and develop a negative perspective. Instead of making the best of a difficult situation, we may bemoan our bad fortune, blaming others and ourselves. Our lives become bogged down. But if you want to blame anyone for life's difficulties, blame Adam and Eve. As we all know, God created a wonderful life for them. All their needs were provided for and they lived in a paradise called the Garden of Eden. They had no financial problems, sickness, war, crime, aging (their life was eternal), or worries of any kind. Their only restriction was that they could not eat from the Tree of Knowledge. Well, along came the serpent, and you know the rest of the story. We have been paying for it ever since. But once you understand that life is hard, it is much easier to keep a positive attitude in the face of life's inevitable adversities.

A second classic is entitled *Man's Search for Meaning,* by Victor Frankel, and is recommended reading for anyone having a tough day. In his book, Frankel chronicles his four years of horror in a Nazi concentration camp. He describes unimaginable conditions, such as marching in the snow with your toes sticking out of your boots and being sustained by a single cup of soup at the end of a grueling day. Frankel recalls inmates regularly losing fingers and toes to frostbite, while having to constantly endure the brutal treatment of the sadistic guards. In this dire condition, Frankel observed the importance of attitude, which he refers to as the last of the human freedoms. Although the Nazis had taken everything from their prisoners, including their property, their quality of life, and their freedom, they could not take away the last of the human freedoms—the ability to choose your attitude despite your circumstances. Frankel noticed that those prisoners who were able to see beyond their immediate misery and focus their attention on a positive goal stood a much better chance of surviving. Some of the goals set included liberty, being reuniting with their family, or even retribution against the brutal Nazi prison guards. But those who didn't set goals and who decided to give up died quickly and easily.

Can you honestly say that any of your current hardships are as difficult as Victor Frankel's were at the Nazi concentration camp? Probably not. He was even tested again at the very end of his horrendous ordeal, as the concentration camps were being liberated. As the Allies advanced on the camp, a rumor spread that the guards planned to kill anyone who remained. The prisoners were given the choice of staying at the camp or departing on a train. Many prisoners panicked and got on the train. Frankel didn't. He kept his perspective at this critical juncture, with freedom in sight. He listened to his instincts, which told him that he survived the camp this long and should therefore remain there. As it turned out, the passengers on the train were the ones who were killed, in a last desperate action by the Nazis. The camp was liberated by the Allies and Frankel lived to tell his amazing story, which stands as a testament to the power of a positive attitude.

We all know people who seem genuinely happy despite leading very difficult lives. Their courage and resiliency are most inspiring. And conversely, there are others who are always complaining despite living in relatively good circumstances. The difference is attitude. One group has chosen to focus on the positive aspects of life and look for the good in challenges and setbacks, while the other is mired in negativity.

My grandmother always remained happy and upbeat despite physical infirmities. As she grew older, her hearing became progressively worse. I would be hoarse after getting off the phone with her. She also broke her hip when she was ninety-three but made a full recovery, as I chronicled earlier. She needed to use a cane but did not seem to mind. She never lost her love of gambling and would meander through the casinos with her cane, oblivious to most of the sounds around her but genuinely happy. When the subject of her hearing would arise, she would simply shrug her shoulders and say that something had to be wrong with her—why not that?

Patience is an important corollary to a good attitude. It can be easy to become discouraged in any new undertaking or even after years of effort. There will always be obstacles. Too often we dream of overnight success, which rarely happens. Instead, history is full of those who tried and tried and it was only later in their careers that they finally experienced great success. I once toured the Liberace Museum in Las Vegas. Although I was never particularly a fan of his, he was certainly a household name when I was growing up. A sentence displayed in the museum humorously stated: "Liberace became an overnight success after twenty years of hard work."

Your attitude affects how you cope with adversity. Psychologists categorize coping behaviors into two types, control oriented and escape oriented. Escape-oriented coping is generally negative and involves being immobilized by a particular setback. Escape-oriented coping includes whining or obsessing over a problem without taking any constructive action. Instead, the person avoids or ignores the problem and even tries to mask it with substance abuse. On the other hand, control-oriented coping is more positive and centered on finding solutions to problems. It involves focusing on the lessons learned from a particular situation and the steps needed to address it. Control-oriented coping and perseverance often go hand in hand. Those who can bounce back from short-term defeats with a new vigor or a new approach can generally press on and ultimately succeed. Resolve to turn challenges into opportunities. Don't dwell on your failures. Learn from them and try again.

Maintaining a positive perspective or attitude often involves striking the right balance between realism and idealism. One needs to be realistic about life challenges but optimistic that they can be addressed. However, taken to its extreme, realism can descend into pessimism or a tendency to imagine the worst. Our feelings and outlook are influenced by our attitude, which filters and interprets all of our life experiences for us. The lens of a negative attitude tends to magnify problems and setbacks while that of a positive attitude yields a more realistic image, which can reduce the problem to a manageable size.

It's easy to have a good attitude when things are going well. But when we are running late, or feeling frustrated or disappointed, or thinking the entire world is conspiring against us, we are challenged to keep our spirits up. Even being stuck in traffic or experiencing car trouble can be a test of your attitude.

Humor can serve as a tremendous boost to the attitude. How many times has a difficult situation been diffused by the use of humor? The gravity of almost any situation can be lightened this way. Somehow things don't seem so bad when you can laugh about them. I read the moving story of a Vietnam POW who spent seven years in captivity. He recounted the horrific conditions of prison camp in Hanoi, nicknamed the Hanoi Hilton. But his suffering was eased for a moment when he took a shower in the squalid conditions and noticed a familiar caption under the faucet: Smile. You're on "Candid Camera."

As we will discuss in the next part of this book, exercise and diet can have a profound effect on your attitude. I know that when I exercise regularly, I have a better attitude throughout the day.

Hurricane Katrina: A Lesson on Perspective

> Anyone can hold the helm when the sea is calm.
> —Publilius Syrus, *Moral Sayings*

> When the levee breaks, I'll have no place to stay.
> —Led Zeppelin

Nothing puts matters in perspective more quickly than a natural disaster, especially if you're directly involved. This happened in my case with Hurricane Katrina, one of the worst natural disasters in the history of the United States. Late on a Friday afternoon, I was tying up some loose ends, a little tired and irritated because social obligations had suddenly arisen for the weekend that were going to distract me from my primary task of polishing this manuscript so that I could send it out to my publisher on Monday. That day at lunch, my colleagues and I had briefly discussed a hurricane in the Gulf of Mexico that had struck the Florida Keys and was expected to curve around and make landfall again in Panama City. It was a passing conversation, and we hoped the hurricane wouldn't disrupt a vessel construction project we were involved in.

I had forgotten this conversation and was trying to finish up my work so I could head to a coffeehouse and edit my manuscript. I then received a phone call that not only quickly changed my perspective but probably my life as well. It was my wife, Karen. The National Weather Service had just issued a new forecast that predicted the hurricane would make landfall near New Orleans. Her office had requested that employees cover their equipment and prepare for the worst. My initial reaction was denial. How could that storm make such a radical change in direction?

I tried to reassure her and told her not to worry. But she replied, "I have a real bad feeling about this. We're due one." I winced, because her intuition was usually accurate.

Was this the Big One?

The greater New Orleans area had been largely spared in recent years, so like everyone else, I had grown a bit complacent. If you've never lived near a coast, chances are you've never had to undergo the harrowing experience of evacuation, which is the stressful task of throwing together your belongings and then heading out of town. The hours prior to a hurricane can be quite frantic, securing personal belongings, boarding up windows, filling bathtubs and containers with water (in case you need it upon returning), and scouring the supermarkets and hardware stores for water, batteries, and nonperishable food items. There is always a general panic in the air as people scurry around making last-minute preparations. Hotel rooms quickly book up near and far, and thousands of people hit the road. Those whose lives were reasonably secure just hours before are driven from their homes as refugees.

Often, mandatory evacuations can come quite suddenly,

requiring painful choices to be made when gathering up belongings. In the case of Hurricane Katrina, I barely had time to take any valuables with me. Usually you grab important papers, family pictures, and other items of sentimental value. I know one family that told each of its children before Katrina to take one thing that was most important to them. Then, before you drive off, you turn and take one last look at your home, hoping against hope that it will remain unharmed.

In the past, most in the area returned to homes fairly close to the conditions in which they were left. There was some yard work to be done, but that was about it. New Orleans hadn't been hit by a major hurricane since Betsy in 1965. I remember that my family had fled to a multistory hotel in the above-sea-level French Quarter and we all huddled in our rooms. Usually the electricity is the first thing to go, and you endure the howling of the winds in the dark (and the heat). Betsy flooded much of the city and resulted in hundreds of deaths. Since Betsy, most of the major storms had missed New Orleans, sometimes just by a whisker. Four years later, Hurricane Camille battered the neighboring Mississippi Gulf Coast with winds close to two hundred miles per hour. The storm surge wiped out much of the coast and killed hundreds, including all but one of the attendees at a well-publicized and deadly hurricane party in a Gulf Coast apartment complex.

There was periodic discussion, especially during height of the hurricane season during the months of August and September, about the Big One, the hurricane that would strike New Orleans from the southeast and dump the lake into the city, much of which is below sea level. There were several recent close calls. In 1992, Hurricane Andrew struck west of New Orleans and inflicted significant damage to coastal areas. In 1998, Hurricane Georges set its sights on the Big Easy but veered at the last minute and struck Mississippi. In 2004, Hurricane Ivan was initially projected to hit New Orleans but came ashore near Gulf Shores and Pensacola. Since I lived on the New Orleans Northshore close to Lake Pontchartrain, I had evacuated for the last two storms. Usually, things returned to normal fairly quickly. Sometimes you lost electricity for a day or two—no big deal.

The Big One? No, things will be fine. Still, I was a bit

anxious as I left work and headed to the coffee shop to edit the manuscript. There was a slight buzz there about the storm, but Katrina's quick change of course had left many hopeful that the unpredictable storm would change course once again.

I arrived at home in time to watch the ten o'clock news. I knew that the area was in serious trouble as soon as the face of longtime weatherman Bob Breck appeared on the screen. His usually bubbly demeanor was replaced with an ashen-gray grimness. He didn't have to say anything. It was the Big One. I watched stunned as he solemnly outlined the storm's projected path along the dreaded cone. The predicted strike zone was relatively small, with all of the models beginning to converge with deadly accuracy. Katrina was headed straight for New Orleans. An evacuation had already been ordered for the low-lying coastal areas.

I left my home around 11:15 that night to fill up my gas tank, so that I would be ready to move the next day. Any remaining doubt about the storm's path was erased by the sure sign of an approaching hurricane: long lines at the gas station. The twenty-four-hour service station was always deserted at this hour. Obviously, others had watched the news and were preparing for a hurricane. I had a bad feeling in the pit of my stomach as I waited in line. This couldn't be happening. Everyone seemed to have a dazed, sullen look on their faces. I exchanged knowing glances with others as I pumped gas. The Big One.

It'll turn, I thought as I went to sleep. But by the time I awakened on Saturday, nearly all of the storm trackers were predicting landfall Monday morning in southeast Louisiana. I spent most of Saturday securing possessions and getting supplies. My neighborhood close to Lake Pontchartrain was subject to mandatory evacuation, with a storm surge of over twenty feet predicted from the lake. My house was raised, but not that much.

While I was preparing, I received an important message on my BlackBerry, a device that would serve as my lifeline in the hectic times after the storm when communication was very difficult. The message was from Louisiana governor Kathleen Blanco's office, stating that she would be convening a conference call at eight o'clock Saturday evening with her department heads and legislators from the affected areas to share information and answer questions. I served in the Louisiana House of Representatives, representing a community on the Northshore of New Orleans. I dialed into the conference call shortly after finishing up around my house. The first person to speak on the call was a representative from the National Weather Service, who stated quite matter-of-factly that a category-4 hurricane—which could grow to a 5—with sustained winds in excess of 145 miles per hour was moving north by northwest at 10 miles per hour and was expected to make landfall directly west of New Orleans Monday morning, placing the city and surrounding areas squarely on the deadly east side of the eye wall of the hurricane. In other words, the Greater New Orleans area had less than forty-eight hours to live. There was a hushed pall afterwards, and then each cabinet member detailed the evacuation plan and the location of storm shelters. The gridlock from the evacuation for Hurricane Ivan had taught the administration a lesson, and there was actually a good contraflow plan with both sides of the interstate leading out of the area and away from danger. The Hurricane Ivan evacuation had been a disaster, with traffic flow reduced to a snail's pace, taking twelve hours to cover the 70-mile distance from New Orleans to Baton Rouge. As it turned out, the Katrina contraflow plan was about the only thing that the state got right for that hurricane.

I doubt that anyone on the call had any idea of the enormous challenges that lay just ahead. I know I didn't. There was no mention of any plan to provide transportation to those who were unable to evacuate, to provide adequate provisions for the New Orleans Convention Center or the Louisiana Superdome, which would served as massive evacuation centers, or to provide the additional security that would be needed to protect citizens before, during, and after the storm. As we would later find out, there was no mention of a plan for these important areas because there was none. A few buses were sent to New Orleans, but they remained parked at the Superdome rather than rounding up people in the neighborhoods. As it turned out, this lack of planning would lead to disastrous circumstances.

The participants of the call were then permitted to ask questions.

A colleague of mine, Rep. Nita Hutter, represented low-lying St. Bernard Parish, which is below New Orleans and would likely be history after Katrina. She tried to sound calm as she requested the phone numbers of the Louisiana State Police and the Louisiana Office of Emergency Preparedness, knowing full well that her constituents would need all the emergency help they could get. I jotted down the numbers also, not realizing how much I would refer to them in the subsequent days and weeks.

I inquired about the routes out of the area that would be alternate to Interstate 10. I knew that many of my constituents would evacuate, and I wanted to be able to give them a useful shortcut out of the region. That turned out to be Highway 190, which runs adjacent to I-10.

There were other questions relating to the evacuation and available resources. One of the last comments was made by Rep. Cedric Richmond, who represented the Ninth Ward of New Orleans. It would turn out to be one of the hardest hit areas of the city, flooded badly by Katrina and then reflooded by Rita. He noted that, in his neighborhood, people were attending baseball games, and they seemed unconcerned about the approaching storm. This lack of urgency bothered him, particularly since the city had not yet called for a major evacuation. His words were prophetic, as many people in New Orleans would choose to stay behind.

A mandatory evacuation was not called until nine o'clock the next morning. It was the first one in the city's history. By then I was on the road to Lafayette. I had left at five o'clock Sunday morning with my family.

We stayed glued to the news for most of Sunday afternoon and night. Some of the weathermen were predicting a turn to the east, which could spare the city, but by Sunday evening, no turn had materialized. A colleague of mine from the legislature called. His parish president was predicting the nightmare scenario—ten feet of water in New Orleans and adjoining parishes and a thirty-foot storm surge that was certain to take my house out. Late that night I dropped to my knees and prayed. The Big One.

I woke up early on Monday morning to amazing news. The storm had in fact shifted to the east and New Orleans would miss a direct hit. An emergency official predicted that the area would be spared major damage. On Monday, we remained glued to the weather channel. Mississippi was obviously being pounded. The news from southeast Louisiana was spotty. Finally there was footage of significant flooding in a suburb of New Orleans. The eastern part of the Northshore was also experiencing significant wind damage. New Orleans was experiencing significant wind damage but was mostly dry.

However, most of the city began filling with eight to ten feet of water due to major breaks in two levees. People there who initially thought they had been spared the worst of it suddenly had to flee to their attics and rooftops as water consumed houses in a matter of minutes. The authorities were totally unprepared. There were not adequate provisions in the evacuation shelters. The electricity had gone out as expected, but the generators that were supposed to run several hospitals went under water and were inoperable. There were literally thousands of people stranded in attics or on rooftops. It was chaos.

The next four days were one of the most agonizing periods of sustained anarchy in our nation's modern history. With law-enforcement personnel overwhelmed by the magnitude of the crisis and the search and rescue operations, criminal elements overran the city. There was widespread looting as well as unspeakable acts being committed in the shelters. Two police officers committed suicide and hundreds fled their posts. As federal assistance lagged, the venerable New Orleans newspaper, the *Times-Picayune,* was reduced to begging with its first headline: *Help us, please.* Yet there were many tales of valor as well as horror. The world stood transfixed as New Orleans seemed like the lost city of Atlantis, only it was sinking into hell.

Two parishes below New Orleans, Plaquemines and St. Bernard, had been virtually wiped out. Thirty-four people in a St. Bernard nursing home drowned. The Mississippi Gulf Coast was particularly devastated, with the towns of Bay St. Louis and Pass Christian virtually wiped off the map. Dockside casinos in Gulfport were blown across the street.

I returned to survey my legislative district, which had extensive damage, seemingly one out of every three houses with a tree on the roof. The Northshore's lakefront was literally destroyed, with steps remaining where one of the houses formerly stood. Although I personally had some flooding damage, many trees fell around my house rather than on it. I shuttled between my district and the Office of Emergency Preparedness to follow through on requests for assistance, including one for 500 military police when order in my area became dicey. With the New Orleans news media entirely knocked out, I used the Baton Rouge media to report on conditions for many of my constituents who had left the area. The anarchy in New Orleans was dominating the news.

I based myself in Baton Rouge so that I could be close to the Louisiana Office of Emergency Preparedness, where much of the hurricane relief effort was being coordinated. The headquarters was bustling with an assortment of representatives from the military, FEMA, government, state police, and media. The criticism was beginning to mount about FEMA's responsiveness, but Michael Brown seemed happy enough as he bounced around the building in khakis and deck shoes. His mild presence was in stark contrast to that of Homeland Security secretary Michael Chertoff, who, with his entourage, rushed through the building in army fatigues, scattering people out of his way.

I hung around for a while, trying to figure out how the system worked, but then I realized that there was no system. With various federal, state, local, and nonprofit agencies involved in a hodgepodge of assistance for immediate needs, the rules were being made up as we went along. Those who seemed to be getting things done were those who were able to collar the right people. But you often had to keep asking around until you found the right person.

Security was becoming a growing concern in my district as our law-enforcement resources were stretched thin. There were reports about the violence in New Orleans spreading to other areas, and we were concerned about it spilling across the lake, which was largely considered a safe haven from crime. There were rumors of isolated looting, and a nurse at a large hospital even reported some rapes in the area. I called the administrator of another local hospital and found out about one rape. A woman in her thirties was attacked while cleaning her house. She had apparently left the door open. There were also reports of a carjacking in a neighboring parish.

I was at the Office of Emergency Preparedness late one

night when the parish requested 500 National Guard troops in addition to generators and other supplies to run our emergency operations. When the formal request came in by fax, I noticed it was given to a state official, who put it in his briefcase to take home. I asked to make a copy and then questioned him about the procedure. He explained that the Office of Homeland Security would order the troops through their "e-system."

"Who puts in the order?" I asked.

"Some guy who sits in the crisis room."

"Where is the crisis room?"

"Third door to the left," he answered.

"Who can request an order?"

"The parish president can."

I pointed at the fax. "Well, didn't he?"

"It needs to be on their letterhead."

It was midnight. "Let me call around," I said.

I tried to get someone at the Parish Office of Emergency Preparedness, but the calls wouldn't go through. I needed to get this order processed. I went to the third door to the left and entered the crisis room, where people were huddled in cubicles and a screen showed news reports and map information. Although it was now well past midnight, the room was alive with activity.

"How do I order 500 National Guard troops for St. Tammany Parish?" I asked.

"You need to make a request on the e-system," one man responded.

I was getting a little weary of this e-system. "Well, how do you make a request?"

"You have to have it typed directly into the system."

I was starting to get really frustrated. *"Who does that?"*

"I do."

OK. Now we were getting somewhere. I showed him the fax.

"It's supposed to be on letterhead from the parish president," he said.

"I know. I can't reach him."

"OK. I'll type it in."

"Thanks."

I leaned over and helped him with the wording as he

typed the order in: "500 National Guard to assist law enforcement with keeping security in St. Tammany Parish."

"I don't want to happen there what happened in New Orleans," I added, but it was not in the order. "Now what do I do?"

"Wait and see what happens," he said.

"Who can expedite this?"

"The White House," he said, adding that he had received a call the day before about snipers in St. Bernard Parish firing on the rescue boats.

I made a mental note to call a contact that I had at the White House. While I was standing there, another public official walked over. He was one of U.S. senator David Vitter's aides, and I asked for his help. He agreed and said that Senator Vitter was fighting to keep some National Guard troops in St. Tammany that someone else wanted to pull. I thanked him and left. It was past 1:00 A.M.

Early the next day, I received a frantic call from a friend of a friend, a computer and networking genius who provided Internet connections and communication services to hospitals in downtown New Orleans. He was hunkered down in a deserted New Orleans office building, dodging looters and running his entire operation on diesel fuel. However, his fuel was almost out, and the lives of patients hung in the balance. Could I get him some diesel fuel? It was the height of the chaos in New Orleans. I told him that I would see what I could do, knowing that I had to do a lot more than that.

I called the emergency headquarters and started asking around. "How do I have diesel fuel delivered?"

"Where do you need it?"

"Downtown New Orleans."

"Oh God, you can't be serious. I don't know how you are going to get fuel out there."

I made a few more calls and finally found the young lady who represented the oil marketers. Her office was close to an evacuation center in Baton Rouge and the police had advised her to leave her office. But she was toughing it out as long as she could.

"Natalie, can you help me get some diesel fuel?"

"Where do you need it?"

"Downtown New Orleans."

"Oh God! I don't know. The driver disappeared on the last truck we sent down."

"Really? What happened?"

"We don't know. We sent him down and that's the last we heard from him."

"I understand, but it's an urgent situation."

She told me to call the agriculture commissioner's office. He was in charge of transporting fuel in emergencies, but the trucks had to be accompanied by National Guard troops.

I called his aide, whom I had known for many years, and the request was put in the queue. I spent the next few hours coordinating delivery, and by the end of the afternoon, the computer whiz had his diesel fuel.

Although things started improving by Friday, the immensity of the catastrophe and devastation was starting to sink in. I had grown up in New Orleans and could not bear to see it turn into a war zone. One million people had evacuated the area. The water stood in the city for weeks and was soon contaminated. The economic impact was unfathomable. Businesses were wiped out along with homes. The port was shut down. Companies began relocating operations. Many of my Northshore constituents worked in New Orleans. Now what would they do? I heard many stories about people leaving the state for good.

Days blended into each other. I was engulfed by family, legislative, and work matters, not to mention trying to clean up my house. Every day seemed to be a battle to restore essential services to my constituents. The heavily wooded Northshore had hundreds of miles of power cables knocked out. Sewerage plants were down. Each day brought a new crisis, from establishing shelters to distributing food, water, and ice. Thousands were left homeless, and all available real estate was quickly gobbled up. I tried to keep my head on straight and do my best, but I knew that my world had forever changed. Within a few days, the area had gone from business as usual to having the economic engine of the state entirely under water. It was beyond comprehension.

But I don't want to neglect the many stories of heroism. One of the more touching interviews I watched on television was that of singer Charmaine Neville, a relative of the famous Neville Brothers, a musical group that truly defines

New Orleans and its Jazz and Heritage Festival. She was being comforted by Archbishop Alfred Hughes and sobbing through her poignant story. She had collected her neighbors when the floodwaters rose and taken refuge on the second story of a school. She cared for her neighbors while trying to wave down rescue helicopters that kept passing overhead. Days went by, and then criminal elements attacked the group. They molested the women, including Ms. Neville. Finally, in desperation, she stole a public transit bus and evacuated the group to Baton Rouge and to safety.

There are many other poignant stories, including that of a man who was holding on to his wife and children, trying to save them from the rushing waters. His wife told him to let go of her and save the children. His last image of her was as she was being pulled away from him by the rushing waters.

Each day I awoke hoping that the whole ordeal was just a nightmare I was having. It tested my resolve to its core. I felt it ironic to be editing a book about the importance of a proper perspective just as my attitude was being sorely tested. So I began to focus on what I could and could not do. As a public official, I needed to concentrate on helping my constituents in the short term while helping to fashion a long-term recovery plan for the area. I focused on the resources being poured into the area and noted that, every day, things became a little better. It will take years to determine how this story ends. But Katrina's devastation not only provided perspective—it challenged my perspective as well.

Things Happen for a Reason

While it's hard to understand a tragedy as horrific as 9/11 or Hurricane Katrina, which is described above, realizing that things happen for a reason can help improve your perspective. This is much easier to understand in the context of smaller setbacks, where there is not enormous loss of life and property damage. There's no point in constantly analyzing or regretting past events. Instead, have faith that certain events occurred for a particular reason you're not aware of yet, and then move on. Perhaps the event taught you a needed lesson, or your desired outcome was simply not meant to be. If you find yourself swimming upstream all the time, it might be time to reassess. You don't want to spend all of your life trying to climb up a particular ladder only to discover it is leaning against the wrong building.

Successes and failures can often be separated by the way they are interpreted. How many times have things turned out differently from your original plans only to end up actually being in your best interest? Adversity can often be a good teacher. Sometimes, unfavorable events continue to happen in your life until you finally learn your lesson. When you experience a setback, dissect the incident. Think of the things you did wrong. Also consider the things you did right but perhaps could have done better. Learn your lesson, but don't obsess over what you did wrong. Otherwise, you might be destined to repeat your mistakes.

It is much more constructive to believe that things happen for a reason than to think you are situated under a dark cloud. Naturally, there is adversity that can be very difficult to understand, such as a death or illness. Sometimes there is no apparent reason for a disaster that we can comprehend. But our reversals seldom rise to the level of catastrophe, though it may seem so at the time.

The general rule is that if you're not going to be bothered about a particular incident one year from now, then it generally falls short of a disaster. Even though it might feel as though the world is ending right then and there, you will probably be able to live through the circumstance. As bad as it might seem at the time, there is generally some reason behind it. It is your choice to either allow day-to-day reversals to darken your outlook or instead use them to sharpen your mind and strengthen your resolve.

During a pressure-packed sporting event, one bad play by an athlete can often lead to a downward spiral in their performance. However, champion athletes are able to shrug off a mistake and come back even stronger. Momentum in athletic events can shift in a single play. The same shifts can occur in your life. It is up to you to decide whether or not you allow a negative event to cause a downward spiral or resolve to regain your momentum.

Many people have turned great adversity into great accomplishments. Think of the late Christopher Reeve, who played Superman in the feature films. He was seriously injured during a riding accident but was able to rebound to serve as a tremendous inspiration. Among other things, he was very active in fund raising for those with spinal-cord injuries.

Mothers Against Drunk Driving (MADD) was also founded after tragedy. In 1980, thirteen-year-old Cari Lightner was killed by a drunk driver in California. The offender had been released on bail for a hit-and-run drunk-driving crash two days prior and had already been convicted twice of drunk driving with a third plea-bargained to "reckless accident." At the time of Cari's death, the offender was carrying a valid California driver's license.

Enraged, Cari's mother, Candace Lightner, and friends gathered at a steakhouse in Sacramento. They discussed forming a group named "MADD—Mothers Against Drunk Driving." Thus, MADD was born with a name that would sweep the nation. Since MADD's inception, alcohol-related traffic fatalities have declined 43 percent. Statistics indicate that in 1980, 55 percent (28,100) of the nation's 51,091 traffic fatalities were alcohol related. In 1999, alcohol-related fatalities represented 38 percent (15,794) of the nation's 41,345 traffic fatalities. Due in large part to MADD's efforts, more than an estimated 138,000 people are alive today.

MADD is an inspiring example of turning tragedy into a positive outcome. Resolve to remain positive and respond constructively to life's setbacks. Learn your lesson, but try to keep the tuition low. Also realize that, on one of those worst days that you can possibly imagine, on those days when everything that could go wrong did go wrong, when you feel as though you are hanging onto a lifeboat and you don't have a friend in the world, if you have your health and your family intact, it wasn't really that bad of a day after all.

Pay Attention

> Life is what happens while you are making other plans.
> —John Lennon

Another important way to maintain a proper perspective is to be diligent and pay attention what's going on around us. We often become so lost in our own little world that we become oblivious and insensitive to the needs of others as well as the lessons offered by the universe. The universe often sends us clues about life that can be easy to overlook if we're not paying attention. If we're not careful, our lives can dribble away while we are making other plans or preparing to do something else.

Be vigilant for signs from the people in your life. Keep your eyes open for those who might need help—a family member who needs some additional attention or even a friend who is in distress. I once heard a touching sermon about helping others by a respected deacon who also runs a food center for the underprivileged. He delivered his sermon just before Christmas and outlined two antidotes for holiday depression. The first was to have faith and the second was to help others. Often we become so impaled by our own problems that we totally ignore the concerns and well-being of others. Why is it thatthose people who seem the happiest are serving others? Do something to make someone else feel good and you will often benefit.

Also pay close attention to the important people and situations in your life. Too often, we see what we want to see and hear what we want to hear. Most of my friends who later divorced told me they were aware of potential problems before they became married. Many didn't listen to the wise counsel of friends and family members and, most importantly, ignored their own doubts and fears. On the flip side, there are those who let their important relationships deteriorate.

So view life positively but realistically. But most of all, pay attention and view life honestly. Extend this honest assessment to all areas of life. Resist the temptation to sugarcoat issues and avoid dealing with them. Admit to yourself when a mate is unsuitable or a job is wrong for you.

Remember the lessons from Adam and Eve mentioned earlier. They essentially forfeited paradise by eating from the Tree of Knowledge. Of course, they were prompted by the serpent to throw away the good life. The bad news is that we live in an imperfect world and we are surrounded by negative influences in our own lives. How many times are things going well and we disrupt the apple cart for no apparent reason? People leave good marriages and good jobs to pursue situations where the grass might appear marginally greener.

We are tempted throughout our lives by negative forces that loom around us. Be vigilant and beware. Often we know what is right and what is wrong but still succumb to the apparent lure. We will discuss negative forces, also known as the enemy, in the spiritual chapter of this book.

The surest way to lose perspective is to compare yourself to others. There is always someone who is better looking, smarter, richer, and more successful than you. If you live your life in the shadow of others, you always feel inferior.

A final important way to maintain a proper perspective is to step back and see the big picture. It's easy to become so immersed in our day-to-day activities that we miss what is truly important. Contrast the "significant" event with another one that effectively dwarfs it, such as an illness or the near miss of a tragedy. Such a close call puts life in perspective. Keep a proper perspective at all times. Our family and our loved ones are much more important than our day-to-day career struggles. Don't wait for something bad to happen before you realize how good the rest of your life is. Keep perspective.

CHAPTER 9

Step 6: Perseverance

Nothing in this world can take the place of persistence. . . .
Persistence and determination alone are omnipotent.

—Calvin Coolidge

Never think that God's delays are God's denials. Hold on;
hold on fast; hold out. Patience is genius.

—Comte de Buffon

(n.) The state or quality of being insistent, bold and defi-
nite in character; obstinately making a stand; persistence.

The final simple step in the tune-up process is perseverance.
The tune-up steps are interrelated as well as integrated, so
much so that you can do the first five steps well and still fail
if you decide to quit too soon. Sometimes we become so
accustomed to instant gratification that we can be easily
deterred by obstacles. But "God's delays are not God's
denials." Still, it can be so tempting to quit and sabotage our
own success. Boomers sometimes have the mistaken attitude
that things are supposed to get better. But life is full of setbacks and pitfalls, and perseverance needs to be the foundation for all important aspects of your life, from saving money,
to advancing your career, to evaluating your life.

Few notable accomplishments are ever made without first
having to overcome setbacks, failures, and bumps in the
road. Most successes have resulted from a dogged and dedicated effort. Perseverance is the glue that holds the other
tune-up steps together.

It is rare for any effort to proceed exactly as planned, despite
careful preparation and the most painstaking attention to
details. The successful person must be able to cope with rejection, overcome "the slings and arrows of outrageous fortune,"
and press on in the face of inevitable setbacks. Just because you

don't win every battle does not mean that you can't ultimately win the war. Treat failure and difficulties as temporary setbacks.

Failure is actually quite relative. In truth, you never fail until you throw in the towel and quit. Persistent people simply keep at it until they succeed. Famed inventor Thomas Edison made a career of failure. He failed 6,000 times before developing the light bulb. When asked how he felt about his numerous false starts, Edison claimed that he didn't fail but simply discovered thousands of ways of how not to invent the light bulb. The key is to learn from your mistakes and persist. During difficult and frustrating times, focus on solving the problems instead of becoming frustrated. You never know as success could be often just one attempt away.

A poignant example of someone who stopped just short of success was author John Kennedy Toole, who wrote the Pulitzer Prize-winning novel *A Confederacy of Dunces*. Since he grew up in my hometown of New Orleans and his book highlighted its unique quirkiness, I took particular interest in the book and, of course, him. Toole wrote the novel while a young man in the 1960s and it might have been a little ahead of its time. He was unsuccessful in having his novel published, despite many attempts. He became deeply despondent and tragically took his own life. However, years after his death, his mother, Thelma, persisted on her son's behalf to have the novel published. She persuaded famed author Walker Percy, who wrote the critically acclaimed novel *The Moviegoer,* to review the manuscript. He was teaching creative writing at Loyola University at the time. Percy reported that Ms. Toole burst into his office one afternoon and tossed a pile of onionskin papers on his desk, informing him that it was a manuscript her son had literally died for and imploring him to review it. Percy stared distastefully at the faded manuscript and decided to read just a few pages to appease her before he rejected it. To his surprise, Percy became quickly captivated by the novel and recommended it to the editor of Louisiana State University Press, who also liked its bizarre humor. A modest first printing was run and the book soon became a cult classic in New Orleans. I found out about it from some of my friends. A few months later, the literary world was turned upside down when the obscure novel that was posthumously published was awarded the Pulitzer Prize for fiction. LSU Press became the first and only university press to win the prestigious prize. The tragic aspect about it all was that the novel was a blockbuster all along, but the author failed to persevere to see its phenomenal success.

A caveat not always found in self-help books is that a good attitude and a game plan don't guarantee success. Many people with grand dreams never achieve them. Many who ran for political office lost despite running great campaigns. Many who started noble ventures were not successful. The path to your dreams will not always be straight. There is often no one around to pat you on the back for trying hard. Simply put, life is not always the linear path to successive grade levels that you became accustomed to during school years. Climbing up life's ladder does not always occur in neat little steps, and consequently you don't always achieve your goals at regular intervals. Progress can often be quite amorphous, with tremendous initial effort exerted but little immediate return. No wonder it's so easy to become discouraged.

That is why persistence is so critical. Many authors' first books are not successful or even published. Sometimes the results from years of writing (as I well know) come much later in life, when all of your effort finally begins to show dividends. Abraham Lincoln remained committed to his path despite tremendous setbacks. He said, "I will study and prepare myself and then one day my time will come." The reason why so few achieve any memorable success is because it is so easy to give up along the way. It takes a great effort to achieve a great result. Those starting a diet have to be diligent for weeks before seeing any results. Then the pounds suddenly start dropping off.

But still enjoy your life and avoid living solely for the payoff at the end. Savor each moment and each step that brings you closer to your dreams. Learn from your failures and don't neglect the important people in your life. No day is lost in which some spiritual truth becomes clear. Accept that life has its inevitable twists and turns.

Persevere and don't give up. Remember the immortal words of one of history's finest leaders, Winston Churchill: "Never give up. Never, never, never give up."

Balance and the Tune-Up Process

CHAPTER 10

Maintaining Balance

Sow a thought, reap an act;
Sow an act, reap a habit;
Sow a habit, reap a character;
Sow a character, reap a destiny.

—Anonymous

Part 2 of this book outlined the tune-up process. In Part 3, we will apply the tune-up process to the following areas of your life:

Emotional
Financial
Career
Relationships
Physical
Mental
Spiritual

Including these important areas within your tune-up plan helps provide the essentials for a balanced life. Too often, hard-driving business executives sacrifice their family and even their health in the sole pursuit of career and financial goals. But even the most distinguished career achievement at the expense of your health and family will end up as quite hollow in the long run. Balance replenishes your power and restores your perspective. Just as missing a tune-up step can send you sprawling, neglecting an important area of your life can leave you unfulfilled and bitter in the end.

Here are a few thoughts about each area of balance.

Emotional balance is essential for your overall well-being and effectiveness. Recent research indicates that your emotional intelligence, or "emotional quotient," can have an even greater impact on your success and happiness than can your IQ, or "intelligence quotient." Maintaining emotional balance can be quite challenging in today's turbulent world. It can be very beneficial to understand and control your emotions. Achieving emotional balance can also be referred to as "getting a grip."

Your financial status affects not only your current lifestyle but also how much or even whether you will enjoy your retirement years. Recent statistics indicate that most baby boomers are not saving enough to adequately fund their retirement. The good news for most of you boomers is that you still have time to accumulate a retirement fund, provided you are willing to sacrifice in the short run and commit to a sound savings and investing plan in the long run. Your goal is to become financially bulletproof, so that you are not dependent on your children, relatives, or the government to fund your golden years.

Your career serves not only as a mechanism for supporting yourself, your family, and your retirement but in many ways helps to define your purpose in life. Since you spend most of your waking hours at work, it is essential to choose a career that you love and that offers you the greatest chance to explore your unique potential. Work will always be work, but if you do work, you might as well be as happy as possible.

But in your quest to succeed, don't allow career and financial goals to overshadow your relationship with the important people in your life. Material success means very little if you don't have special people in your life to share it with, which includes your spouse, children, other family members, and close personal friends who add meaning and enrichment to your life.

Personal health is one area of life we take for granted until we lose it. The sad fact is that most serious medical conditions, such as heart disease, diabetes, and even cancer, are lifestyle related and can be prevented. Despite having the best health care available in the world, the health of our population continues to deteriorate. Record numbers of people are now considered obese and neglect their bodies. Proper exercise and diet can provide enormous benefits to both the quality and quantity of your life. Not only can they reduce stress and extend our lives, but they can provide a sorely needed break from our daily grind.

Another way to battle the aging process is to keep your mind sharp. Never lose your intellectual curiosity. There is always something new to learn or discover, which helps keep you from stagnating. All successful people have a passion and a drive for learning. Also, flood your mind with uplifting and enriching thoughts. You do tend to become what you think about most.

A regular spiritual practice can greatly assist in centering us and maintaining clarity about those aspects of our lives that are truly important. A good spiritual foundation empowers us to make better decisions and lead more effective lives as well as find that often elusive sense of inner peace. Too often, we only turn to God when all else fails. Don't wait until you're at the end of your rope to reach out for the healing power of spirituality. Incorporate a regular spiritual practice into your day-to-day activities and watch your life become calmer, clearer, and more focused.

As you examine each of the important areas of your life, draw an imaginary line in the ground between your old habits and thoughts and the new life you wish to lead. Don't let self-defeating behaviors drag you backwards. Forget the past and don't become distracted by regret. View all your experiences as necessary for your progress. Learn from your mistakes, but don't dwell on them. The "if only" list can be endless and will consume us if we let it. If I have any regret at this point in my life, it is that I spent too much precious time consumed in worry and distracted by regret. We are so prone to torment ourselves. If only I had pursued another career, saved more money, made better investments, or married someone else, then . . . Then what? Everything would be fine, or would it? Maybe, but then again maybe not. But as much as we'd sometimes like to, we can't go back and redo our lives. By lamenting your past, you sabotage your future. So forget your mistakes and missed opportunities and concentrate on *now.*

CHAPTER 11

Emotional Tune-Up

Never let yourself be driven by impatience or anger. One always regrets having followed the first dictates of his emotions.
—Marshal de-Belle-Isle, letter to his son

Let every man be swift to hear, slow to speak, slow to wrath.
—James 1:19

No one can make you feel inferior without your consent.
—Eleanor Roosevelt, *This Is My Story*

The *Oxford English Dictionary* defines the term "emotion" as "any agitation or disturbance of mind, feeling, passion; any vehement or excited mental state." According to the book entitled *Emotional Intelligence,* "emotion" is "a feeling and its distinctive thoughts, psychological and biological states, and range of propensities to act."

As humans, we have both a rational mind, which is based upon our mental thought processes, and an emotional mind, which is triggered by our emotions. But unfortunately for us, our emotional mind usually works more quickly and more powerfully than our rational mind and can harm us if we let it. It is essential to understand and control your emotions, or they could end up controlling you. The classic example the reaction to being cut off on the freeway by a discourteous driver. Although your rational mind might suggest that you put this incident behind you and move on, you become really angry or worse yet stay mad all day and take it out on your co-workers or family.

Primary emotions include anger, sadness, fear, enjoyment, love, surprise, disgust, and shame. Emotions such as sadness or fear can be painful to experience. But they are natural emotions and can be very appropriate in certain situations.

Sadness is natural upon the death of a loved one, and fear can actually be useful in threatening situations. It is natural to be fearful while traveling in a bad neighborhood, and your heightened vigilance could actually help protect you. However, if you are still fearful after the danger has passed, then the emotion serves no particular use. Fear, in particular, can serve to stifle your dreams and aspirations. Anger is another emotion that can negatively affect your quality of life. Some people become easily enraged over some insult or discourteous behavior, and their anger can often exceed the situation. However, controlling your emotions doesn't necessarily mean blocking them out. You still want to "feel" or experience your emotions.

If I had a dollar for every time a therapist asked a client, "How do you feel?" I would be quite wealthy. That's because many people in therapy have difficulty "feeling" or "expressing" their emotions. Their emotions either bottle up inside and cause internal havoc or eventually boil over into rage.

The term "emotional intelligence," or "emotional quotient (EQ)," refers to how well people handle their own emotions. Achieving a "high EQ" involves the following:

- *Identifying and labeling feelings.* The first step to a higher emotional intelligence is identifying and understanding your feelings. Hence the favorite question of therapists. Suppose you don't feel quite right. Are you sad? Angry? What are you sad or angry about? If you are able to identify and understand your feelings, then you are better able to address them.

- *Expressing feelings.* The flip side of allowing your feelings to control you is the inability to express your feelings. Expressing feelings such as love is critical in interpersonal relationships, particularly with family members. It is also important to express other emotions when appropriate.

- *Assessing the intensity of feelings.* This skill allows us to be more proportionate in our emotional response to different situations. Are we deathly afraid of a particular situation? Are we becoming too angry over little things? Fear or anger can easily debilitate our lives if we let them.

- *Delaying gratification.* One of the strongest human impulses is the desire for gratification. As a society, we have become very accustomed to instant gratification.

But the ability to delay gratification is an essential life skill.

- *Controlling impulses.* The emotional tug of impulses can be quite intense. A comment or action can prompt an irresistible need to respond. We pass a store window and are suddenly purchasing something beyond our means. But our ability to control such impulses can improve our quality of life as well as our chances for success.
- *Reducing stress.* Stress is cumulative, and our complicated, fast-paced society can literally overwhelm us if we let it. Most illness is stress related and, left unchecked, stress can destroy us.

Although it is obvious that emotional health is a critical ingredient of our well-being, actually managing our emotions can be quite challenging. Highly educated and trained professionals, such as psychiatrists, psychologists, and other licensed therapists, spend their entire careers trying to help people understand and control their emotions. But even for these professionals, "fixing" their patients is not as easy as putting a crown on a tooth or removing a ruptured appendix. I have friends who have been in therapy for years or who keep bouncing from one emotional disaster to another. Sometimes their self-destructive emotional patterns are quite obvious. They keep changing careers or spouses in an effort to feel better. Others hate the status quo but are afraid to even consider a change. They instead remain in a state of perpetual gloom and doom, frozen by worry that is often grossly out of proportion to reality. Still, emotional fixes are not always easy, and I am far from fixed myself, despite a great deal of work. Also I'm not claiming that this book can necessarily fix you, but it certainly can help.

You can dramatically improve your emotional state and your life by honestly evaluating yourself, assessing your emotional state, and then making the necessary changes. Often, people find the last step most difficult. It is easy to receive advice but often hard to implement it.

Once I found myself regularly confiding in a friend about my consuming bouts of anxiety and sluggishness that were paralyzing me every morning and that I couldn't seem to shake. She listened politely a few times before offering some profound counsel: "Maybe if you started working out again in the morning, you'd feel better."

I protested that her simple solution ignored the severity of my hardships and said there was simply no way I could follow her advice. I was too busy in the morning, and besides, how could I possibly even think about exercise when I felt so bad to begin with?

She was undeterred. "Maybe if you started working out again in the morning, you'd feel better." She also reinforced her advice by calling me every morning to coax me out of the house and off to the gym.

Eventually, I resumed my morning exercise ritual and, eventually, began to feel much better. My problems were still there but my debilitating anxiety wasn't. Sometimes the solution to emotional difficulties can be quite simple.

So why did a treadmill and some free weights make such a difference in my life? From a physical standpoint, the activity released endorphins into my system, which trimmed stress and supplied energy. We will discuss the benefits of a physical tune-up in a later chapter. The workout also provided a sense of accomplishment and the perfect pad from which to launch my workday. And I enjoyed renewing acquaintances with the morning regulars. But most importantly, my morning routine forced me to start moving instead of wallowing in my troubles. Although I absolutely hated getting out of bed to face the predawn chill, my discipline was rewarded with a more comfortable emotional state.

Emotional issues challenge us every day. Advances in technology and health care have done little to control our day-to-day stress.. If anything, our wireless society, with its cell phones and Internet-enabled personal digital assistants, has kept us more connected to the sources of stress as opposed to providing convenience. Our health-care system is more focused on treating the effects of emotional disorder, such as heart disease and high blood pressure, than on reducing its root causes. Emotional problems can range from common neurotic tendencies to profound personality disorders. Chemical imbalances in the body can also contribute to emotional distress.

The good news is that most of us do not have severe emotional problems. Although we all have emotional impediments to our happiness and well-being, they can be addressed to a large extent, provided we make the effort. Whether you wish to seek professional counseling is up to you and the depth of your problems. I have benefited tremendously from professional counseling but have also been helped by my own research and advice from wise friends. The insights into our psyches that provide the breakthroughs for emotional growth can come from a multitude of sources, provided we are willing to keep digging and pay attention. Although we may not outgrow all of the hang-ups and complexes of our youth, we don't have to be ruled by them.

Emotional Baggage Obstructs Passion

We start our lives overflowing with passion. Watch how newborns marvel at the world around them. They are fearless bundles of energy, tumbling and exploring with reckless abandon. Small children remain filled with a lust for life as they play energetically and boldly with their friends.

I remember visiting my niece's first-grade class. Their teacher mentioned that they had all just finished an artwork project and asked who wanted to show theirs to the visitor. The students rushed to display their work. I compared their reaction to some of the adults I have taught at a college level. Unlike the children, adults often cringe when they are asked to share their ideas. Somewhere between the time we are born and the time we become adults, our passion becomes obstructed, often by the self-consciousness of adolescence or even sooner.

As we journey down the river of life, our emotional baggage is floating all around us. Some pieces drift away while others can stick to us like flotsam and jetsam. We start collecting our baggage quite early and innocently. Perhaps we were teased as children or embarrassed by a thoughtless teacher. Other refuse can be created in our early years by our parents, grandparents, siblings, and other relatives, who often exert a tremendous influence on our development. Psychologists sometimes refer to such emotional baggage as "family of origin" issues. Such issues could have been created in an "at-risk family system," which included compulsive behavior by one or more parents, such as alcoholism, gambling, or even an obsession with perfection or achievement. I mentioned earlier that I grew up in an alcoholic household, which is apparently so common that there is even a name for people like me: Adult Children of Alcoholics ("ACOA"). According to the literature in the area, ACOA generally have problems with intimacy, commitment, and substance abuse. That struck a familiar enough chord with me to open my eyes and start me on my arduous path to recovery. I shudder to think where I could have ended up otherwise.

Emotional baggage can be quite subtle. If a frog is tossed into a pot of boiling water, it will quickly try to hop out. However, if the same frog is placed in a pot of water that is slowly heated, it will not realize the danger of the gradually increasing temperature until it is quite cooked.

What part of your past could be reaching the boiling point? Childhood experiences can be much more insidious than you realize. I have a friend who is obsessed with her weight. Despite being a beautiful woman with an enviable figure, she is so dissatisfied with her appearance that she actually hates her body. This unhappiness has spilled over to other areas of her life. As we talked about it, she mentioned that a close relative often ridiculed overweight people while she was growing up. This insight helped her to realize the source of her self-consciousness. In addition, I once read of a very humiliating childhood incident of a small boy who was forced by his father to play basketball. He was skinny, uncoordinated, and rarely played. Once he was sent in late in a particular game and ran eagerly onto the court, with his slight frame and his skinny legs. As he stood on the court, everyone in the gym started to laugh. It should be no surprise that to this day, he hates sports, particularly basketball.

Other demons from the past include those from an emotionally shocked family system, such as divorce, chronic physical illness, abandonment, violence, or death. Your family could have been rigid about traditions or practices. Other problems could have included boundary violations such as emotional, physical, or even sexual abuse.

All families are dysfunctional to some extent, and the lingering effects can range from mild fears and neuroses to deep traumas and pain. In addition, all of us have had to pass through the pain of adolescence, which teaches us to be overly self-conscious. Our bodies suddenly begin changing, and we can often mature physically more rapidly than we do emotionally. This awkward phase can create issues and fears that plague us in later years.

"Codependent" became a popular buzzword in the 1990s. Psychologists define this as a pattern of painful dependency on compulsive behaviors and on approval from others in an attempt to find safety, net worth, and identity. Codependency is a common family of origin issue.

By the time we reach midlife, we have all accumulated our share of emotional baggage. Sometimes we are not quite sure what is wrong. We could be burdened with a general sense of sadness or even self-defeating behaviors that can imprison us and prevent us from living life to its fullest. Our psyche might feel riddled with holes, causing us to feel incomplete and miserable, seeking attention. This can drive us to alcohol, gambling, or other addictions for relief. We try to deaden our feelings, but our emotional pain can envelop us like a straitjacket, wringing out our quality of life drop by drop. When our emotional wiring is faulty, we compromise not only our passion for living but also our most important and intuitive gauge for life—namely our feelings. Excessive emotional baggage can leave us constantly distracted by dealing with our pain as opposed to living our life.

The process of ridding yourself of emotional baggage is called recovery. The purpose of recovery is to understand the source of your emotional pain and then begin to address it. Recovery begins when you reframe your thinking and look for the positive aspects of your life or even the divine protection that has insulated you from even further difficulty. Part of the recovery process involves reconnecting to your feelings, or passion, even if it makes you emotionally vulnerable. As recovery continues, you may stop avoiding risk and change and feel empowered enough to act on your feelings. The recovery process also enables you to nurture yourself and begin to experience and recover your passion.

Embracing your feelings is no easy task. Often, a major step includes the removal of self-destructive behaviors that were used to mask or medicate your uncomfortable feelings, such substance abuse. Many mistakenly turn to alcohol, drugs, and other compulsive behaviors to create passion or even peace in their lives. Although I am not a Big Book-thumping AA proponent, I do believe that there is a considerable amount of substance abuse and other compulsive behaviors affecting this country.

I have attended twelve-step meetings for ACOA, in which I have heard stories of alcoholism burning through a family tree like a forest fire. Sometimes the disease (and alcoholism is a disease) skipped one generation, only to reignite at the next one. I have heard families tearfully recount the devastating effect of alcohol and other substances on their parents, grandparents, and even their children. My hometown of New Orleans boasts a robust drinking culture. Although there is nothing wrong with having a good time, substance abuse can destroy lives—directly, by the impact of the addiction, and indirectly, by masking deeper emotional issues. It is virtually impossible to address the underlying emotional issues, which could sabotage your recovery, unless you handle any substance abuse issues in your own life.

My father's drinking had a significant detrimental effect on my childhood and young adulthood. My relationship with him had been strained over the years and had always been a source of pain and regret in my life. I never could understand why he apparently neglected his family in favor of his barroom buddies. I would sometimes call him at work to find out when he was coming home. He would assure me that he was on his way and I would sit outside and wait for him in the front yard. Usually, he wouldn't show. Maybe he intended to come all along but became sidetracked by a call from one of his drinking buddies. Maybe he decided to just stop for a short one that turned into a long one. In any event, he would not show up for dinner, usually rolling in well after midnight, and I would be awakened by the loud, vicious argument that inevitably ensued.

As in many households, our troubles were simply not talked about. My parents even became upset when they found my journal describing the chaos. How dare I call into question the peace and tranquility of our family! My father was not alcoholic, I was told; he simply liked to "relax" with his friends. He was a man's man. Alcoholics were people who could not hold their liquor, became intoxicated on one drink, drank alone, or consumed hard liquor, all of which conveniently did not apply to my father. He only drank beer in barrooms with friends as a recreational activity.

The real tragedy was that my father was generally a good person. People really liked him and he was loyal to his friends. However, eventually his alcoholism took complete control of him. His career spiraled downwards, and he lost his business and his family and—to some degree—his soul.

I could never understand why my father chose the barroom over his family until I began to address my own recovery. Many years later, after his marriage to my mother had ended and while I was still trying to maintain some semblance of a relationship with him, I reluctantly agreed to accompany him on Father's Day to his favorite bar. He walked from my car to the bar with his usual shuffle, his head down and his body swaying from side to side. But his posture changed dramatically when he hit the front door of the bar. He cocked back his shoulders in a military posture as he strutted confidently into the bar with his adult son in tow. As my eyes adjusted to the darkness, it seemed our entrance was duly noted by all of the barroom patrons, who were spending a beautiful Father's Day Sunday afternoon in the dirty, window-less tavern, drowning away their lives. As my father slid easily onto a stool, the bartender placed a bottle of beer before him without asking. Although he insisted that I "have a drink with my pa," I still ordered a soda. One by one, he began introducing to the bar patrons his son, the corporate attorney who worked for the big Fortune 500 company. They had all obviously heard of me (probably more than they wanted to) and I shyly nodded my greetings.

It was then that I finally understood my father. The barroom was his passion, the only place he felt comfortable and whole, the corner joint where everyone knew his name. The alcohol and the esteem of his drinking cronies filled his holes better than the love and companionship of his family. His passion and his life had been totally overtaken by his addiction.

In order to recover my own passion, I had to confront any substance issues in my own life. Since alcohol had never interfered with my studies or work, I mistakenly believed that it was not an issue for me. But as I immersed myself in books about self-help and spiritual growth, I realized that children of alcoholics have a high predisposition to becoming dependent on alcohol themselves.

A spiritual experience finally helped me address this important issue in my life. Often, spiritual insight can be an important component of emotional recovery. During a religious retreat, I was led to the decision that I simply wasn't going to let alcohol jeopardize my life. The risks were too great.

So consider whether there are any chemical dependency issues in your life. If you're not sure, then consult with a professional. Generally, if you're a little worried about substance abuse in your life, there's reason to be. Don't let drinking or other compulsive behaviors such as gambling, promiscuity, shopping, or even eating disorders block your passion and ruin your life. If you're experiencing problems with any addictive behavior, or any loved one has ever confronted you with them, please get help.

Although simple in theory, the process of recovering our passion can be difficult in practice and often takes years to fully achieve. For most, the process of recovery is a lifelong journey. However, remember that this seemingly endless journey begins with a single step. Recovering your passion is the first step to emotional well-being.

Make Emotional Well-Being Your Purpose

> Nothing gives one person so much advantage over another
> as to remain always cool and unruffled under all circumstances.
> —Thomas Jefferson

Earlier we discussed taking charge of your emotional health and ridding yourself of your clutter piece by piece. I have seen many people, including myself, make amazing strides in improving the quality of their lives simply by deciding to examine their emotional wiring.

Unlike physical health, emotional health can be considerably harder to measure. People do not schedule annual emotional checkups each year, as they do physical checkups. And unfortunately, many don't even schedule physical checkups. In addition, the symptoms of emotional distress can be more subtle than those of a physical illness, although emotional conditions can be related to a physical condition, such as depression or a chemical imbalance.

In other words, emotional wellness cannot necessarily be examined by a stethoscope. A good indication of emotional wellness is the ability to control emotions as opposed to being controlled by them. Individuals with this ability are slow to anger and generally handle crises very well. They usually get along well with others and don't react disproportionately to frustrations in their lives. They seem balanced and unruffled, handle stress well, and generally have an optimistic outlook.

Part of an emotional tune-up is learning how to manage your emotions effectively. Emotional health involves locating this control internally. If you don't take your emotional wellness into your own hands, you will be continually sidetracked by outside events that "push your buttons" and control your state of mind. Taking charge of your emotional health can help heal you, help you understand some of your emotional triggers, allow you to experience your feelings, and, more importantly, allow you to fully enjoy your life.

The purpose of the emotional tune-up is to enhance emotional health and maturity, so that your emotions are not short-circuiting the other areas of your life. Emotional wholeness is evidenced by the ability to constructively handle or even embrace your pain. There is much pain in life, much of which is caused by fear. Many of our fears, such as fear of change, fear of being alone, and fear of the unknown, are triggered from deep inside us. Recovery allows us to understand and address these triggers. By allowing them to linger on, we compromise our emotional wellness.

I have included in Appendix B some of the books that helped me address emotional issues in my life. The classic *You Can Heal Your Life,* by Louise Hay, is a great book for addressing past emotional issues and "healing your life." On the other end of the spectrum, *Emotional Intelligence* is a logical, factual guide to understanding and managing your emotions. *Your Erroneous Zones* and subsequent works by Wayne Dyer combine humor, psychology, and practical wisdom for comprehending and controlling your emotions.

Weekend retreats sponsored by churches and other service groups can help you understand and address many life issues, which inevitably includes your emotional baggage. Much of the spiritual advice imparted at religious services provides guidance on addressing negative emotions, such as depression. In addition to masses, I attend weekly prayer breakfasts sponsored by Pastor Steve Robinson of the Church of the King. He often devotes a multipart weekly series to such topics as fear and stress, recognizing that emotional wellness is important for the congregation.

The tune-up process can provide synergistic benefits, with one area helping another. For example, the financial tune-up, discussed later, can help relieve emotional concerns about finances. The physical tune-up can help you feel better and more capable of handling stress. And, of course, the spiritual tune-up provides the proper spiritual foundation to enlist God's help in your daily journey.

One inexpensive way to launch the emotional wellness process is to join a support group, which can range from church- and community-sponsored groups, to individual Bible studies, to twelve-step programs. Often, the interaction with others in similar situations and facing similar issues helps you cope with life's inevitable challenges. Such fellowship can be important as you tend to your emotional wellness and stability.

The twelve-step programs are based upon the twelve steps of AA, which has a tremendous success rate in curing alcoholics. The twelve-step process combines spiritual values with practical wisdom and provides a blueprint for recovery from past traumas, addictions, and other afflictions. I was assisted tremendously by attending meetings of ACOA, which focused on the fallout of growing up in an alcoholic household. I not only learned a great deal about addiction and living with addiction but also about finding serenity in this tumultuous world.

Although it takes a bit of courage to wander into one of the meetings, the benefits can be tremendous. There are twelve-step programs for practically every condition. The best known is AA, which has probably helped more people stop drinking than any other program. Another group, Al-Anon, helps people cope with problem drinkers in their lives. There are groups to help survivors of incest or domestic abuse, narcotics addicts, overeaters, , gamblers, and people with other compulsive behaviors. These meetings are very inexpensive, as little as one dollar per meeting, and they can provide a tremendous benefit. The key is to shop around and find a group that you are comfortable with. All of them are well intentioned, but in my experience, each group tends to have its own dynamics and chemistry. They meet in the morning and afternoon and on weekends. No one is required to talk or "share," and it is often best just to listen in the beginning. The meetings are always run professionally and follow certain guidelines in order to make everyone feel comfortable. The attendees are there to support and not criticize others.

Another step to improve emotional health is to seek counseling. Emotional issues can be quite complex and often defy blanket remedies. If you cannot work out the distress and unhappiness in your life on your own, it could be helpful to consult with a counselor. In addition to professional therapists, counselors are available through many church organizations. There should be no more stigmas attached to visiting a mental-health professional if you are not feeling "right" emotionally than to visiting a doctor if you are not feeling good physically. I view a counselor as I would a personal fitness trainer: someone who can help coach you into a desired state of emotional wellness, provided that you are willing to do much of the heavy lifting yourself.

Many seek professional counseling when they hit the proverbial midlife crisis. Trained professionals can help their clients sort through the traumas and difficulties in their lives and guide them towards a path of recovery or emotional wellness. Many family of origin problems were disguised in the Ozzie and Harriet generation that characterized post World War II family life. Back then, it was simply not fashionable to talk about substance abuse or other troubling issues. Instead, they were swept under the rug. The advent of self-help literature in the 1980s and 1990s opened the eyes of a whole new generation to the recovery process, using such terms as "codependency" and "the dysfunctional family." John Bradshaw wrote and widely lectured on reclaiming your "inner child" and the positive impact of re-parenting yourself. His popularity demonstrated that many people were struggling with painful family of origin issues.

Professional therapy can help you pinpoint and address patterns of behavior and unresolved issues that can subconsciously undermine your decision-making process and influence your response to certain situations as well as cause you pain and grief. We all know individuals who can't keep jobs, who go from one bad relationship to another, and whose lives generally are in disarray. In most cases, their emotional wiring is faulty. Such internal wiring is generally subconscious and often has its roots in childhood experiences. Therapy can help you address these often unconsciousness and self-destructive behaviors that cause you pain and discomfort and lead to poor choices in your life.

Following is list of considerations in selecting a professional therapist:

1. Are they addiction/compulsion free? If not, are they in an active recovery program?
2. Have they received specific codependency training?
3. Have they received specific experiential therapy training?
4. Are they supportive of twelve-step programs?
5. Do they support the concept of alcoholism as a disease?
6. With whom do they work best?
7. Where, when, and to whom do they refer clients?
8. How will you know when you are finished with them?
9. Is there evidence of a sense of humor?
10. Do you feel comfortable and safe with them?
11. Do they have access to a full range of feelings?
12. Can they both support and confront?
13. Do they show healthy self-worth and are they consistent and dependable?
14. Are they respectful?
15. Do they set clear boundaries about time, fees, missed appointments, and client responsibility?

Sometimes it is helpful to ask others to refer a therapist. Deciding to consult with a therapist is a very personal issue and should not be taken lightly. As in any profession, there are good therapists and bad therapists. However, finding the right one can be a key to unlocking significant emotional pain. It was for me.

Trained professionals can also help with the chemical imbalances that cause depression and other debilitating mental conditions. Although I believe such medicine should be administered judiciously, it is appropriate in certain cases. So if you have some lingering bad feelings that you can't shake, consider consulting with a trained professional.

Forgiveness

Let not the sun go down on your wrath.

—Eph. 4:26

Always forgive your enemies; nothing annoys them so much.

—Oscar Wilde

Forgiveness is perhaps the most important lesson for reaching emotional wellness. So often, we doggedly hang onto resentments and bad feelings and spend considerable energy lugging them around with us. We never realize the true weight of such bitterness and its negative impact on out emotional health. Why not let it go? I have friends who can recite verbatim all of the wrongs that were committed against them. Before I came to understand the power of forgiveness, I could criticize my father for hours on end to anyone who cared or even didn't care to listen. I have discussed emotional baggage that is accumulated from childhood and young adulthood. However, it is important to realize that your parents did the best they could, and you should forgive them completely for issues you might attribute to them. I also had difficulty forgiving my first love, who, quite frankly, could be pretty mean at times. We dated again when I was in law school. For some reason, I couldn't forget her high-school slights. She would try to explain, through a bewildered barrage of tears, that she was young and immature at the time and would ask why I had to keep bringing it up. We eventually broke up again.

I was also adept at holding grudges against others. It seemed that no matter where I worked, someone would always get under my skin. I would memorize their offensive behavior and could rant on about it at a moment's notice. Once when I was complaining (again) about a co-worker, my mother pointed out that I always seemed to be upset about someone I worked with. Indignant, I disagreed and argued that my charges were more than justified. But the more we talked, the more I realized there was coincidentally at least one antagonist in my life at all times. Many of the people who had previously given me fits were long gone, yet I still wasted so much time and energy on them. I finally realized that life wasn't sending me enemies—I was creating them myself. Although these individuals could be difficult at times, I was the one empowering them to control my life. We all come across our share of difficult people, but they only become antagonists if we let them.

There will always be those who are unkind and inconsiderate. But if you wait for everyone in your life to act properly, then you may be waiting a long time. There are always those who talk badly about others, refuse to wait their turn, and do other things to intentionally disrupt your life. But that doesn't mean you have to react in kind. If someone wrongs you, let it go. I'm not saying to become a doormat, but don't hold on to every grudge. It's just not worth it. Resentment and anger can consume you if you let it. So what if you're right? Do you want to be right or be happy? Too many people make themselves miserable by insisting on being right.

It is so tempting to assume the worst motives when we become angry with someone. We think people are out to get us and their offensive behavior is intentional and mean spirited. But even the most malicious people have some redeeming qualities. Maybe they are just having a bad day. Maybe they are generally insecure and unhappy to begin with. Perhaps that is why they are lashing out at the world. Remember that you're not perfect either, and there are two sides to every situation. Empathy, or understanding another's point of view, is an important hallmark of emotional maturity. So avoid being too sensitive and learn to let things roll off your back. I remember the scene from the movie *On Golden Pond* when actress Jane Fonda was complaining to her mother, played by Katharine Hepburn, about her difficult and ill-tempered father, who was of course played by her real-life father, Henry Fonda. Hepburn made a very memorable reply. "Sometimes you have to look real hard to realize that a person is doing the best that they can." Don't forget to look real hard before judging someone.

Still, forgiving is not always easy, and my father presented a formidable challenge in this area. For much of my life, I carried tremendous resentment against him. His drinking had disrupted our family and caused significant financial problems. Although just out of law school, I had guaranteed the refinancing of my family's house so that we would not lose it by foreclosure to my father's business debts. I also moved back home "temporarily" to help pay the bills, while he tried to straighten out the family finances. But as time passed, none of my father's supposed deals materialized, and his absences from home were becoming more frequent. My "temporary" return home was becoming an extended stay. I had always hoped that my law degree would be my exit visa from the family whirlpool, but it apparently wasn't enough.

Finally, on one crisp Sunday morning, I broke. It had been a horrendous week. I had gotten skewered in my annual performance review at the law firm the previous week. I knew my family pressures were at least partially to blame. And I couldn't even share my plight with my family since I was sort of the breadwinner. To make matters worse, the previous night my girlfriend had admitted that her recent business convention in Hawaii had included a male traveling companion. I was actually more upset at myself for being so naive than I was with her. That Sunday morning, my father and I were sitting alone at the breakfast table. He was reading the newspaper and I was staring listlessly out of the window. Although the day was off to a bright, promising start, all I could sense was darkness. Finally, I couldn't take it anymore. I confessed to him my frustration that my hard-earned professional paychecks were being gobbled up by household expenses. I had studied hard and worked my way through school. Wasn't that enough? I didn't deserve this. My father tried to calm me down, cautioning that my mother might hear us and cause an even bigger scene for him to deal with. But I kept on, insisting that I just couldn't take it anymore and pleading for him to help out some. He placed his hands on my shoulders and assured me that everything would be just fine, that he was on the verge of a large real-estate deal that would fund a substantial payment on the house. I would be able to move back to my condominium, and he promised that one day he would pay me back fully. In fact, he had an important meeting that afternoon and might even have some good news by the end of the day. I finally began to see a glimmer of hope.

That afternoon I was washing my car when he drove up. Our house had a long driveway, with a horseshoe drive closer to the street. From the moment my father stepped from his car, I could tell that he was very intoxicated. He literally staggered out of his car and careened up the driveway like a ricocheting pinball. I was stunned. As he walked past, I searched his eyes for an explanation. He avoided my gaze and instead thrust his hands downwards as if to say, "I give up."

I gave up too. I realized that it was all a lie, that everything he told me about his real-estate deal and his supposed work was a lie. In a sense, he was a lie.

My bitterness towards him was eating me alive. Fortunately, I happened upon an audio tape by noted self-help author Dr.

Wayne Dyer shortly afterwards. On it, Dyer recounted a moving story about forgiving his own father. His father had abandoned the family while Dyer was very young, and all that he knew of his father was an abominable history that was only whispered about. He felt the tremendous ache of unresolved feelings. Dyer was miraculously able to locate his father's gravesite on a business trip. In an emotional scene, Dyer expressed all of his unresolved feelings and forgave his father posthumously at the cemetery. This act of forgiveness turned Dyer's life around, and he began his best-selling book, *Your Erroneous Zones*, the very next week.

I was listening to this tape while driving and had to pull over. There was too much of a parallel to my own situation for this to be a coincidence. I realized that I needed to forgive my father. It was very difficult at first. But as I learned about alcoholism, I better understood that his reckless behavior was caused by a progressive disease that destroys anything in its way. The substance abuser feeds the addiction at the expense of everything else. That's why my father's drinking buddies meant so much to him. They were an integral part of his addiction, and his family was not. But why couldn't he see what was happening? Why didn't he at least try to seek treatment? I couldn't say. But he was controlled by forces stronger than himself, and I needed to forgive him.

I later learned that my dad's own father suffered from both alcoholism and depression. Back then, there weren't any medications to treat depression and people who acted strangely were simply put away somewhere. My grandfather was institutionalized when my father was very young. His family faced tremendous hardship and I can only imagine the intense stigma of mental illness in his tough Irish Channel neighborhood in New Orleans. Sometimes he and his mother and siblings would visit my grandfather on Sundays and occasionally bring a picnic lunch. One day he received a phone call, when he was around ten, that his father had passed away.

His mother struggled heroically to hold the family together and did a remarkable job under the circumstances. My father and his brother both served their country in the military, finished college, married nice ladies, and started families. Their sister also married well and it appeared that a happy ending was in store after a difficult childhood. But both of the men had ticking substance-abuse time bombs inside of them and it wasn't long before the bombs detonated, quickly ruining my uncle in the prime of his career but destroying my father more slowly and methodically.

My forgiveness was put to the ultimate test when my father was diagnosed with lung cancer and needed to be taken care of. Unfortunately, cigarette smoking was another of his vices. Although he was closer to my sister, she had her hands full with a husband and three children. I decided to move him from his apartment to my house so that I could take care of him. I drove him to his treatments, and my father faced his illness very courageously and without complaint. I also scurried around trying to assist him with vitamins, experimental drugs, and vitamin C drips. I even tried to cook healthy for him, even though I had little experience in the kitchen. On my third attempt to grill fish one night, he proclaimed that my food was worse than chemotherapy.

It was a trying year, but I was determined to do my best. He was naturally very depressed and we never did have the "talk." I didn't see the purpose of rehashing his life, settling accounts, or even forgiving him in person. I simply wanted him to know that I loved him and I was there for him. I often told him that I loved him, even though he could not bring himself to reciprocate. I knew that he did and I was grateful to be able to share his final year. I came to know him as a very gentle and decent person. He faced death with dignity, and I not only forgave him but came to deeply respect as well as love him. I realized that he was a kind person who was bested by two diseases—alcoholism and cancer. I am finally liberated from all of the anguish and feel completely a peace with my father. But it all began with a willingness to forgive.

I once heard a very poignant story about a woman who was estranged from her biological father. He and her mother had split up when she was very young. There were bad feelings involved and he was never even discussed around the house. He made no effort to contact her. But one day when she was in her early thirties, she received a phone call from his attorney, informing her quite matter-of-factly that her father had passed away and had left instructions to tell her that he'd always loved her. The attorney further explained that the reason he did not try to contact her was because he was afraid of her rejection. She was visibly sad as she recounted the story, lamenting that she would have been happy to visit him had he asked. The fact that she never knew her father had always been a source of pain. She would have gladly forgiven him had she been given the opportunity.

Since then, I have been a staunch believer in the power of forgiveness. I once participated in a year-long recovery program that was facilitated by two licensed counselors. All of the other members of the group were highly functional despite having many families of origin issues as well as substance abuse problems. The group consisted of successful physicians, nurses, attorneys, educators, and homemakers. During the group process, members recounted horrific incidents in their lives, many of which involved their parents. Almost all of the group members were still very angry at their parents, even after many years.

Despite the depressing stories, I preached forgiveness. I urged the group members to pardon their parents' cruelty and neglect. In doing so, I locked horns with one of the counselors, who felt that such blanket absolution trivialized the members' legitimate feelings. In other words, the group members had a right to be upset about their upbringings. The counselor had been abandoned by her own father at a young age and was still very angry about it. But I felt just as strongly about forgiveness and continue to promote it. There were some terse exchanges between us. However, by the end of the program, I had picked up an unexpected convert. At our closure exercise, we sat in a circle and passed a bean-bag around. Comments were offered to the group member holding the bean bag. When the bag reached me, this counselor was the last to speak. She noted that she had fought me all year over the issue of forgiving our parents. But after careful reflection, she conceded in front of the entire group that I was right and she was wrong. We do need to forgive our parents. I was pleasantly surprised by her concession. It requires just as much courage to admit that you're wrong as it does to forgive.

In addition to forgiving your parents, as well as others who might have wronged you, it is just as important to learn to forgive yourself. We spend far too much time berating ourselves about past choices. We agonize over our careers or spouses and fret over roads not taken. Forgiving yourself can be the most difficult task. But you can't forgive yourself until you forgive the others around you. And once you take this important step, your goal of emotional wellness becomes considerably closer.

Empower Yourself Emotionally

The most important battles fought are the battles of the mind."

—Anonymous

The techniques discussed above are methods to empower yourself emotionally. Believe that any emotional issues are within your control and that you have the power to effectively address them.

Emotional empowerment involves stepping back and recognizing the self-defeating behaviors that may have limited you in the past. Methods of emotional empowerment include self-awareness, self-discipline, and empathy. Although our emotional programming is configured at childhood, we still upgrade and even reconfigure our internal software. We can also nurture and strengthen our emotional core, by such techniques as identifying, labeling, and managing feelings; delaying gratification; controlling impulses; and reducing stress.

An important skill for emotional empowerment is managing your self-talk. Self-talk is that little voice inside of you that often chatters incessantly. Such inner dialogue can be a way to cope with challenges and reinforce your behavior but can also cause hardship by constantly berating you. Learn to harness your little voice and speak to yourself in a more constructive dialogue. Like for many others, my own self-talk was extremely critical and served as a constant distraction in my life. The key to controlling self-talk is to simply to take control. We all control our own thought process. Those who appear happy, despite many hardships, have chosen to focus on the positive parts of their lives. Conversely, those who are miserable, despite having many advantages, have become fixated on the negative. We can control our thoughts with self-talk. Instead of giving yourself negative messages, try positive ones.

One potent form of positive self-talk is affirmations, which help to promote positive feelings and awareness. Remember the Stewart Smalley episodes on "Saturday Night Live" that parodied positive self-talk? ("I'm good enough. I'm smart enough. And darn it, people like me.") However, the effectiveness of positive self-talk is no joke. You can make a dramatic impact on your emotional state by simply changing your inner dialogue. There are even products on the market that assist you to create your own affirmations.

Another essential emotional skill is reading and interpreting social cues. Visualize how you fit in a larger context of others by recognizing the influence of your behavior on others and keeping yourself in perspective in the larger community. Often, we become so wrapped up in our own crisis du jour that we ignore the perspective of others. Although it can be healthy to vent anger and frustration, it should not be done in a way that harms others.

This leads us to the importance of understanding the perspective of others. It is very tempting to see the world solely from our own eyes. However, it can be very enlightening to experience another person's a point of view. Once we are aware of the opinion or position of another, it can help diffuse our anger with a particular situation. Instead of berating someone whom you perceive is giving you a hard time, see them as just another human, who is struggling to get through the day. This skill of understanding others is known as empathy. The more you can understand others, the more you can control your own emotions.

Another component of emotional empowerment is developing a realistic expectation about yourself. I often saddled myself with unrealistic expectations, and I was constantly scrambling to hurdle the higher bar. So, while it is important to set goals for yourself, be realistic. Otherwise, you are setting yourself up for failure and constant self-criticism.

Another skill includes self-awareness, which is the ability to recognize a particular emotion and experience it. Such self-awareness requires that you be in touch with your true feelings. The first step in managing an emotion is to be able to evaluate the emotion. Next is the ability to control the emotion. The more you can regulate and control negative emotions such as anxiety, anger, and sadness, the better you will feel and the more productive you will be. One technique is known as reframing, which involves recasting a potentially negative situation in a more positive light. We tend to magnify our problems, obsessing about the worst possible consequences. It is far better to treat every difficult situation as a learning experience that will ultimately be of benefit in the long run. Meditation and prayer can be very helpful in regulating negative emotions. Exercising or taking a long walk can also be of great benefit.

Emotional Tune-Up Plan

> Advice is like castor oil—easy enough to give but difficult to take.
>
> —Anonymous

Assessment. The first step in any emotional tune-up plan is to assess your current emotional state. Be totally honest with yourself regarding whether or not you have substance-abuse or emotional issues. Sometimes professional help and even some close friends can help you uncover any problems in this area. For whatever reason, people paper over many emotional issues that they do not want to face.

Your emotional issues could consist of a lingering sadness or a feeling of unease. But unresolved issues will eventually rear their ugly heads. They usually do not go away on their own but instead need to be addressed. The good news is that there is a great deal of help out there for those who are willing to seek it out. As I mentioned earlier, in addition to professional counselors there are twelve-step programs for almost any condition. Today, there is more knowledge about treating such conditions with programs that work. Take advantage of the constructive ways to combat the negative forces in our lives, which include fear, compulsive behavior, lack of focus, lack of discipline, and lack of understanding.

Deep-seated traumas and insecurities can sabotage your efforts. As I mentioned, professional counseling can assist a great deal in uncovering self-defeating behavior and pain and can send one down the path to emotional well-being. Since much of our emotional health is subconscious, a trained eye and insight can provide tremendous benefits. I have included some of the self-help books I found most beneficial in Appendix B. Remember that tuning yourself up emotionally is something that you constantly have to work at.

I ran the gamut in dealing with my own emotional issues. As I mentioned earlier, I have sat on several couches, spent two weeks in a sweat box bleeding out any impurities, meditated on the beautiful rocks of Sedona, Arizona, and attended countless self-help events and workshops. I find that reaching emotional maturity is similar to peeling an onion. Each layer that you peel provides some insight into past behaviors that have caused you pain. Sometimes these insights come rather quickly; others require more work. I'm not saying that therapists are for everyone. Often, a sympathetic friend can give you the feedback and affirmation that you could get from a trained therapist. Sometimes people end up paying good money just to be listened to.

Everyone has different emotional baggage and different requirements for mental health. If you had an extremely dysfunctional childhood, you might need professional help. Some emotional conditions are chemical in nature and can be treated by medicine prescribed by a physician.

Planning. Once you have made an assessment, the next step is to fashion your plan for emotional recovery. Your plan could consist of the following:

1. Read the books suggested in Appendix B.
2. Forgive everyone, in writing, for what they did.
3. Journal regularly, both to understand and express emotions.
4. Evaluate any destructive behavior and take steps to end it.
5. If you have a particular issue, investigate the twelve-step programs in your area.
6. Engage in stress-reducing activities, such as exercise, recreation, and regular spiritual practice, which are discussed later in this book.
7. Decide to see a counselor if you feel it is appropriate, and do your homework to find the right one.

The goal of an emotional tune-up is to feel good emotionally. If you don't feel good, resolve to undertake a plan that will help you reach your desired state.

Maintaining a Healthy Emotional Perspective

> Those who cannot remember the past are condemned to repeat it.
>
> —George Santayana, *The Life of Reason*

Attitude. This word appears in self-help books more than any other. Most difficulties can be overcome with a positive attitude or a healthy emotional perspective.

As we discussed earlier, we are directly responsible for all of our own thoughts. Those with a positive attitude and controlled behaviors have a much better chance of withstanding difficulties than those with a negative attitude. It is easy to be happy when things are going well. A healthy emotional perspective involves maintaining a proper attitude no matter what the circumstances.

Maintaining a healthy emotional perspective entails flowing with the currents of life instead of fighting them, living in a state of comfort as opposed to discomfort. As we will discuss later, regular spiritual practice can be very important in maintaining a healthy emotional perspective. In today's complicated and challenging world, it is often soothing to "let go and let God." Turn your life over to God and let God make the major choices.

I have found that when I struggled, my life became a struggle. When I accepted events, my life was a lot easier. Such acceptance involves appreciating and celebrating each aspect of life. My grandmother lived very simply during her ninety-nine years and was always upbeat. Even just before her death, when she was very sick, she still got up and got dressed on my birthday.

The Information Age has brought with it a host of gadgets to improve productivity. Although the Digital Age, with its e-mail and personal digital assistants, is dramatically raising productivity, much can be said for simplifying your life and going back to basics. Simplifying involves removing all of the clutter from your life and examining your commitments. Our lives can get very complicated by middle age. We've got all sorts of stuff and mental images and ideas, and part of the tune-up process is paring down the baggage. Many of the burdens in our lives are self-imposed. We rush around gathering things and wind up on the same treadmill each day. It is amazing that, during one of the most affluent times in our society, there is actually such a poverty of quality time. This all suggests that we return to a simple time, a simple life, to clear the clutter and focus on the things that are important.

Life Lessons for a
Healthy Emotional Perspective

Good order makes men bold, and confusion, cowards.
—Niccolo di Bernardo Machiavelli, *The Art of War*

The psychic development of the individual is a short repetition of the course of development of the race.
—Sigmund Freud

Following is a summary of some lessons I have learned for maintaining a healthy emotional perspective:

1. You are responsible for your life. As much as you might like to lay the blame on someone else, the bottom line is that you are responsible for everything in your life.
2. You are in charge of your life. You can't necessarily have everything you want, but you can have just about anything you want. However, success does come with a price. Determine what you want and the price you are willing to pay for it.
3. We all have our share of difficult breaks, but we can always point to people who have had it much worse. Chances are that any setback you have been confronted with has also been faced by others.
4. Address imperfections and self-defeating behavior. We all have some of these that hold us back to some extent. Many of us are held back by fear and remain trapped in our comfort zone. Although everyone experiences such negative emotions, those who are successful are able to address them and overcome self-limiting tendencies. Such control-oriented coping helps to minimize your limitations and maximize your advantages.
5. Success depends largely upon how you handle failure. We are all going to have stresses and reversals in our lives.

Any successful person can point to past failures in their life. Resolve to bounce back and learn from failure.

6. Forgive everyone who ever wronged you. This is important spiritual as well as practical advice. How often do we carry around grudges and bad feelings towards others that only sap our focus and energy? These can be based on petty offenses on up to serious damage that may have been inflicted on you, including by your parents. Remember that your parents did the best they could with what they knew.

7. Forgive yourself. You are not quite finished with forgiveness until you have forgiven yourself. Don't keep badgering yourself for what you perceive as wrong choices in your mate, career, education, or place of residence. God has an unlimited capacity to forgive you, so why can't you forgive yourself?

8. Have patience. God's delays are not necessarily God's denials. In an era of instant gratification, it is particularly important to have patience.

Persevere with Your Emotional Tune-Up

Endure and persist; this pain will turn to your good.
—Ovid

Maintaining a healthy emotional state can be very difficult. The next time you feel bad about something, look inside yourself and see what are the root causes. Resolve to address each underlying issue and focus on emotional wholeness. If you persevere, you can have a tremendously joyful life to look forward to. And when everything seems to be at its worst, persevere and keep your emotions in check.

CHAPTER 12

Financial Tune-Up

The love of money is the root of all evil.

—1 Tim. 6:10

People who make money often make mistakes, and even have major setbacks, but they believe they will eventually prosper, and they see every setback as a lesson to be applied in their move towards success.

—Jerry Gillies, author of *Moneylove*

The more you love what you are doing, the more successful it will be for you. . . . What you do is more important than how much you make, and how you feel about it is more important than what you do.

—Jerry Gillies

Prosperity Consciousness Provides Passion

Prosperity consciousness helps provide the passion for a financial tune-up by regarding finances from a standpoint of abundance rather than scarcity. A belief of scarcity or shortage places you on the defensive, with the fear that there is not enough to go around and that life is a continual financial struggle. We all have financial challenges and make mistakes, but dwelling on them is not going to bring us one step closer to financial security. Instead, develop a passion for prosperity by firmly believing that you can become financially independent. We all know people who have problems with money, those who never seem to have enough or are always spending beyond their means. Money seems to burn a hole in their pockets and maybe yours as well. I read a story about a lottery winner who spent all of her millions in just a few short years. When interviewed about her financial fiasco, she claimed that she just couldn't handle money. She was uncomfortable with it, so she spent it all. Consequently, the first step to financial independence is to become comfortable with money.

Judging by the low savings rates of boomers, many do seem to be uncomfortable with money and therefore they spend it. Others may be intimidated by the confusing myriad of financial products in the marketplace or spooked by past investment mistakes. In addition, the media focuses on the top tier of wealth, giving little attention to average people trying to meet their financial goals. Also, many so-called "sources" of financial advice are actually more interested in selling you something than helping you. In the midst of it all, we are constantly bombarded by advertisers trying to separate us from our money. Striking a happy medium between being a free spender and the proverbial miser involves realistically and prudently managing your money. Many have become financially independent with minimal resources and education. Although prosperity involves some discipline and planning, it is available to those who seek it. Those who attain financial independence have become comfortable with money as well as their ability to manage it. Approaching your finances from the standpoint of self-denial and fear can yield the same disappointing result as a crash diet. Many view budgeting their money with the same disdain as a strict diet—no fun, no frills, just plenty of self-denial. But saving merely means paying yourself first. I call this *Top-Down Budgeting*. Just as passing on desserts and unhealthy food can boost your health and self-esteem, small financial choices can yield tremendous returns later on. The road to financial independence involves a conscious decision to seek prosperity with a fiscally responsible lifestyle. Can you honestly say that you enjoyed items you really couldn't afford? But such fiscal responsibility is more than just working for your money and saving; it is also planning a diversified investment strategy to make your money work for you.

While working as a waiter in college, I befriended a retired attorney who was a frequent patron of the restaurant. He had founded one of the oldest and most prestigious law firms in New Orleans and enjoyed a national reputation in maritime law. As an aside, he was a classmate of legendary Louisiana governor Huey Long at Tulane Law School and actually helped tutor Long for the Louisiana bar exam. His success placed him at the top of the city's social and business elite. He lived in an exclusive Uptown neighborhood and belonged to all of the prestigious social clubs and Mardi Gras organizations. But despite his success and affluent lifestyle, his financial outlook was based more on scarcity than prosperity. Two things happened during his lifetime to shape his outlook: the enactment of the federal income tax and the Great Depression, which was largely caused by the stock-market crash in 1929. As a result, the attorney's entire investment strategy was shaped by his aversion to market risk and income taxes. Upon retirement, he liquidated his assets and placed them in tax-free bonds. These assets included not only real estate and stocks but 100 original paintings by John James Audubon. Although retirement is certainly a time to remove some risk from your investment strategy, my lawyer friend went a little overboard. He shielded himself from market decline and taxes, but his very conservative strategy left little room for his assets to appreciate or work for him. Worse yet, his static holdings provided little protection against the double-digit inflation of the 1970s, which brutally chipped away at his net worth.

Actually, I didn't really know his financial situation until he passed away and his family requested that I handle the estate. My great-uncle had died at around the same time and I was preparing his succession as well. I was startled to discover that Uncle George's estate was actually larger than the prominent attorney's. Uncle George had never attended college and owned a small furniture store. His income was modest, probably a fraction of the attorney's. But my uncle's portfolio was more diverse and included stocks and bonds, real estate, and ownership in several small banks in the area. Time had been on my uncle's side, because his money had worked for him. On the contrary, time had been the attorney's enemy and had eaten away at his life savings.

In addition to making your money work for you, it is important to learn to pay yourself first. This seems rather basic, but savings rates in this country have fallen to all-time lows, particularly among baby boomers. Those of us who were born in the decades just after World War II were fortunate to have grown up amidst tremendous prosperity. The war had devastated Europe and there was huge demand for U.S. services and products. We naturally assumed that things could only get better. Therefore, many of us do not observe

sound saving and investment principles in our own households. My family, for instance, lived beyond its means. Not all
of the spending was frivolous, since it included education
and family vacation expenses. But it still placed an enormous
burden on my father, and this pressure may have con-
tributed to his problems.

Many Americans are approaching midlife with an
uneasy feeling about their finances. However, don't panic,
because there is still time to shore up any financial weak
spots, provided that you're willing to put the prosperity principles to work. Financial security is within your grasp if you
are willing to go after it. Know that despite an ominous stack
of bills, a checkbook that never seems to balance, tax returns
that are due, and a paycheck that never seems able to stretch
far enough, things will eventually work out if you commit
yourself to a prudent saving and investment plan.

Make Financial Independence Your Purpose

Everyone wants financial independence. However, fewer
than 5 percent of Americans will become financially independent. The good news is that you can be one of them if
you're willing to take the necessary steps now.

As for any goal in life, financial independence requires
discipline as well as a proactive attitude. Financial security
will not necessarily come to you—you have to earn it. It's not
about winning the lottery, finding the big deal, or discovering the killer business idea. Rather, it is based on accumulating wealth slowly and methodically, through a systemized
approach of saving and investing.

As we discussed above, the simplest way to save is to pay
yourself first, the Top-Down approach. Most people pay
themselves last or save whatever is left over after all the bills
are paid—the Bottom-Up approach, which in many cases
doesn't add up to much. Paying yourself last instead of first
can make it difficult to fulfill your purpose of financial
independence. That is why deferred savings plans such as a
401(k) can be so helpful, because people become used to paying themselves first. Many companies match your payments,
which can provide an even greater return. In addition,
Congress has provided tremendous incentives for these
programs by making contributions and gains tax free or, in

the case of Roth accounts, making gains and qualified distributions from the account tax free. I have prepared many wills over the years and noticed that personal wealth is often concentrated in the personal residence as well as tax-free savings plans.

The next best thing to a using a tax-advantaged account is setting up some type of savings or investment withdrawal with a mutual-fund company that automatically debits your checking account. Again, this forces savings to come off of the top. Buying an investment asset, such as real estate, is another way to force savings.

Prosperity consciousness does not have to be all work and no play. According to the book *The Millionaire Mind,* those who achieve great wealth are often well rounded and quite normal. They love their chosen vocations and are able to balance their financial goals with an enjoyable lifestyle. The authors, who studied millionaires quite closely, found a positive correlation between the number of activities people took part in and their net worth. In other words, those who achieved wealth were active in the community, coming into contact with others who later become clients, customers, suppliers, patients, or just friends.

Don't confuse prosperity consciousness with greed. The term *greed* took on a new meaning in the movie *Wall Street,* when Academy Award-winning actor Michael Douglas, playing the obsessed takeover artist Gordon Gekko, proclaimed that most memorable line that "greed is good!" The purpose of financial independence is to accumulate sufficient resources to enjoy a comfortable retirement without depending on outside parties.

In fact, greed led many, including myself, to get burned on the stock market. We were not greedy in the sense of avarice but in the sense that we lost sight of financial fundamentals. It simply became too easy to make money with a rising stock market, as people overallocated their portfolios into risky investments.

Financial prosperity is much more about discipline than greed. A certain amount of discipline is required to plan and follow through on your investment strategy. By failing to plan, many people are planning to fail. During the recent market meltdown, many took financial cover, simply refusing to open their brokerage statements.

Another step in achieving your purpose of financial independence is adequately addressing and insuring against possible risks, which could jeopardize your nest egg. Another term for this process is becoming financially bulletproof. This extends beyond simply having enough money to retire on to saving for medical care and long-term care, for example. It also requires adequately addressing your insurance needs and not leaving a "hole in the boat." Such an oversight could undermine your otherwise best-laid plans. My own great-aunt worked hard over the years, never married, and spent most of her life socking away money. She denied herself many simple pleasures in life and became almost obsessed with accumulating savings. She lived to the ripe old age of 101, actually living in three different centuries. However, she required around-the-clock care for the last three years of her life. She went through her entire savings to pay for it. Although it was certainly her choice to spend her last years in the comfort and familiarity of her home, it seemed like such a waste, as she could have easily preserved the value of her estate with long-term care insurance.

The moral of the story is that failure to adequately insure, particularly in the case of long-term care, could send any purpose for financial independence quickly out the window.

Empower Yourself Financially

The next step along the road to financial independence is to empower yourself financially. Another way to consider this is to become financially literate, by empowering yourself with the discipline, knowledge, and resources to fulfill your purpose.

Discipline

Discipline is required for financial independence. It is very easy to part with our money. We often fall prey to buying without thinking. We don't read the fine print. We don't ask questions. We don't comparison shop. And we don't say no. A little bit of discipline in purchasing decisions can go a long way. Take the time to ensure that you receive sufficient value for every purchase with your hard-earned money.

In *The Millionaire Next Door,* which preceded *The Millionaire Mind,* the authors studied millionaires and discovered that most came from average backgrounds. Generally, their financial success resulted from their ability to save more than they spent, which, as you know, is not always easy. Companies spend millions and millions of dollars on advertising campaigns, trying to coax the money out of your pocket. It seems that almost everywhere you turn, someone else is trying to sell you something. To borrow the phrase from the anti-drug campaign, learn to "just say no." Have the discipline to choose your purchases wisely and within your Top-Down budget.

An important corollary to financial discipline is to beware of credit cards, a.k.a. plastic heroin. Some credit counselors recommend that we refrain from using credit cards altogether and instead to rely on a debit card from our bank account. There is an explosion of consumer credit debt in this country. Credit cards can suck the unwary in over their heads before they know it. The reason why you are bombarded with so many credit cards in the mail is that the credit-card companies are making a lot of money on the high-interest payments, even after they factor in the defaults.

Knowledge

The second way to empower yourself financially is through the knowledge of fundamental financial principles. I have many friends who constantly lament how terrible they are with money. Most are intelligent people, some even with advanced degrees. Still, they avoid reviewing their brokerage accounts or otherwise "messing" with money because it's too hard or it makes them feel uneasy. Although, as discussed later, it is important to obtain competent professional assistance, it is equally important to achieve some degree of financial literacy so that you can take a more active part in planning for your own financial future. Such knowledge includes familiarity with basic financial principles, so that you can assess your financial posture, talk intelligently with financial professionals, and assist in your own financial decision-making process.

The reason why so many of us suffered during the stock-market declines of the last few years is because we lost track of the financial fundamentals. If this includes you, don't feel bad, because you are certainly in good company. As I mentioned earlier, my MBA didn't prevent me from following a poor diversification strategy. Below are some important financial principles.

Cash flow. Cash flow is also the "bottom line." Most of our cash flow comes from our salaries and investments. Without adequate cash flow, we cannot sustain ourselves during our career and retirement. Cash flow is also an important medium by which to judge any type of investment opportunity. We generally want to maintain adequate cash flow and need to plan around expenses such as taxes, which can serve as a drain on cash flow. Cash flow is of course the starting point for your budgeting process.

Risk and return ratio. There is a direct relationship between risk and return. Generally, the higher the risk, the greater the return. At the low end of the risk-return ratio are the very secure investments, such as CDs and bonds backed by the government, which have fairly modest returns. On the other end of the risk-return spectrum are more speculative investments, such as growth stocks in startup companies with little or even no operating history. There are many such companies in the technology sector, and they have the potential to produce huge returns. We all know that a single dollar invested in Microsoft in the 1980s could be worth thousands today. That is why Bill Gates is the richest person in the world. However, for every Microsoft, there are thousands of technology companies that did not perform nearly as well. Most investments fall somewhere between government bonds and technology startups on the risk-return scale. These include stocks from more established companies, which are less volatile. Your investment strategy is generally adjusted according to your tolerance for risk. Your personal risk-return ratio is a function of not only your personal preference for risk but also your financial tolerance for risk. Generally, the younger you are, the higher the percentage of your portfolio that should be in equity investments, because your earning capacity and long-term investment horizon are different from those of someone closer to retirement.

Investment vehicles. It is also important to be generally aware of the various types of investment vehicles in the market.

- Common stocks. These are direct investments in equity ownership of the company. Each share of common stock represents a share of the earnings and future growth of the particular company and entitles its owner to a certain percentage of the dividends that company pays as well as the ability to vote on those items that corporate law requires to be approved by the shareholders. That is why you receive those pesky packets with the ballots inside to elect directors and approve other items. Many factors determine the value of common stock, most notably the earning capacity of the company and its future prospects. Other items include the condition of the particular industry, quality of management, projections for future growth, and general state of the economy. There are analysts who follow major companies very carefully, scrutinizing and judging these factors. That is why posting good numbers or exceeding analysts' expectations can cause a spike in a company's stock price. One of the most common factors stock analysts look at is what is known as a multiple of earnings. The market price of the stock per share divided by its earnings per share is known as its multiple, or P/E ratio. This ratio can be very important because it indicates whether or not a stock is overvalued in relation to the market or the overall industry. Generally stocks trade at ten to twenty times their earnings per share. Obviously, earnings are a crucial number in evaluating the price of a stock. That is why companies such as Enron and WorldCom did illegal things to manipulate earnings and prop up their stock price.

  During periods of what former Federal Reserve Board chairman Alan Greenspan described as irrational exuberance, market prices strayed significantly from reasonable price-earnings ratios, going as high as 50 or 100 or even off the charts for companies without any earnings at all. For the long-term investor, the key is to find companies that are solid, with good management teams and a consistent performance history.

- Mutual funds. These consist of collections of securities that are managed by an investment professional. When you buy shares of a mutual fund, you are indirectly buying the shares of common stocks owned by the mutual-fund managers. A common mistake when investing in several mutual funds is to become overallocated in a particular market sector without knowing it. We will later discuss diversification and the importance of maintaining a diversified investment portfolio. Although you might think you're diversifying your risk by buying mutual funds, check carefully to ensure that your funds are not buying the same stocks. Also be aware of the annual fees of each mutual fund, its front- and back-end loads, and the amount of money required to start investing in a particular mutual fund. Sometimes it is better to invest in a family of mutual funds and stay within that family, as they allow you to invest periodically or switch mutual funds.

- Bonds. These are long-term debt obligations of either a corporation or governmental entity that are issued to the general public. The advantage of some government bonds is that they are tax free and have the full faith and credit of the governmental entity. Bonds generally pay higher interest rates than savings and even some CDs at banks. Bond values fluctuate with interest rates but not to the extent that common stocks do. However, bonds are not immune from risk. For example, high-yield bonds can be called in by the company when rates drop. Generally during times of inflation and rising interest rates, the value of the bond will decrease because the interest rates on other instruments are higher.

- Precious metals. These can be good investments during times of uncertainty. Precious metals such as gold, silver, and platinum tend to increase in value during times of economic uncertainty because they are considered to be more stable.

- Real estate. In some markets, real estate has turned into a very hot investment. Real estate can be invested in direct-ly, by buying either rental property or shares of real-estate investment trusts, which generally hold larger properties. Again, careful consideration must be given to real-estate investment trusts, including their track record and man-agement fees. Real estate can be an excellent way to hedge your portfolio, and many have done well with this investment vehicle. However, real estate is not without its downside and is subject to changes in market value. Like anything, the investment market is cyclical and real estate can become quite sensitive to local economic trends.

- Annuities. These are an agreement to pay a fixed sum of money for a period of time in exchange for a lump-sum investment. Annuities can be valuable for retirees and others who want to guarantee a certain percentage and certain amount of income.

Time horizon. A Harvard study shows that the people who were most successful invested for the long term. It is very difficult to predict the stock market, even for the "experts." There are simply too many psychological factors and other variables underlying the market. Therefore, establish a long-term strategy based upon your risk profile and investment choices, and stick to it. Such a long-term investment strategy requires constant discipline, investing during down markets and selling stocks you might like but think have reached their peak. Obviously, those focused on short-term investments will not achieve the same financial security as those looking twenty or thirty years down the road. When I was in college, I managed an apartment building, and collecting rent from its working-class tenants was always a chore. I remember that Friday paydays inevitably led to people splurging on pizza and beer and otherwise blowing their paychecks. It was sometimes a struggle to get the rent money out of the tenants before they spent it. Many of us are not that much better, spending money before we quite have it. Don't think of $100 that you spend today as $100 that you'll make up soon. Think of it as $100 that, invested properly over fifteen to twenty years, could become several thousand dollars. This is viewing dollars with a long-term outlook.

Constant dollar averaging. This is an important corollary to long-term investment. Since it is very difficult to predict the market, it helps to invest on a regular basis. This approach can insulate you from frequent fluctuations of the market. That is why people can be so shocked at the increase in value of their 401(k) plan—money is invested on a monthly basis. A person who invests regularly performs better in the long run than does the sporadic investor. Many mutual-fund investments and even some stock investments allow you to have money debited from your account on a monthly basis for the purpose of making more investments. That helps to automate your savings and investment strategy.

Professional Advisors

The final way to empower yourself is to surround yourself with good advisors. The financial-services industry is in a constant state of flux, and many former insurance salesmen and stockbrokers are now popping up as financial planners. Key financial advisors include a financial planner, a certified public accountant, an insurance professional, and an attorney. The financial planner should prepare your blueprint for financial independence. This would consist of a recommended asset-allocation formula, including a realistic return projected over a number of years to arrive at a final value of your portfolio. Look for someone who is certified as a financial planner (a CFP) or even a certified public accountant who does financial planning. Usually, fee-based financial planners are more objective in designing a financial strategy, since they are less likely to steer you towards investments with higher commission rates for them. The amount of money necessary to have a professionally managed plan has dropped considerably in recent years.

A good investment advisor can be critical to your plan. Some advisors invest in individual stocks, while others prefer a more institutional approach. The right investment professional can empower you in your quest for financial independence and address the myriad issues involved in a financial plan. When choosing a financial professional, it is helpful to understand that there are inherent conflicts of interest in the industry. For instance, stockbrokers at a particular brokerage house can receive additional commissions or incentives for selling certain securities. This hardly makes for an objective investment advisor. It is important to have an investment advisor you trust, because they hold the keys to your financial security. My investment advisor meets with me on a regular basis and provides me with a binder of information, including investment outlook, detailed information about recommended investments, my portfolio allocation, and my projected returns. And he charges no commissions, just an advisory fee.

My investment advisor is also very decisive. I learned the importance of this several years ago, when I was rolling over a substantial 401(k) into an IRA. I set up a meeting with a broker I had used before. He prepared an investment plan for me and told me he felt the timing to buy stocks was quite good, as the experts felt that the market was at or near a bottom and it was down substantially that morning. But before he executed any trades, he suggested that we got to lunch. It turned out to be the costliest lunch I have ever eaten. Between the time we left and the time we returned, the market had shifted dramatically, actually going up several hundred points and thousands of dollars. I suppose the moral of the story is to do your business first and then go to lunch!

In addition to getting a financial planner, find a good CPA to help you structure your affairs to minimize taxes. Also, an insurance professional will guard you against potential risks to your financial well-being, including costs associated with long-term care. Finally, an attorney can handle your estate planning and prepare your will and other documents to put your legal affairs in order.

When choosing your advisors, ask them for referrals from clients, check to see if the advisors are qualified in their specialty, and don't be bashful in talking about price. Be especially wary of noncertified, nontraditional professionals, such as credit counselors. An entire industry has risen around credit counseling and there is considerable abuse in this area.

The key is to surround yourself with people who are not only good at what they do but also worthy of your trust.

Establishing a Financial Plan

> Neither a borrower nor a lender be;
> For loan oft loses both itself and friend,
> And borrowing dulls the edge of husbandry.
> —Shakespeare

> He that wants money, means, and content, is without three good friends.
> —Shakespeare

A plan for financial independence does not have to be complicated. You only need a simple roadmap from your present net worth to your retirement years. This involves answering the three main questions below.

1. Where are you? Calculate your current net worth by determining your assets and then subtracting your liabilities. Either your CPA or your financial planner can help you determine your current financial condition.

2. How much do you need to get where you want to go? In other words, how much money will you need during your retirement years? You will have to project what your health-care and other expenses might be in your senior years. Are there any special expenses with children that you may be responsible for? If you have young children, what about their educational expenses? How much do you need to live, and what kind of lifestyle do you anticipate? Do you desire sufficient disposable income to pay for travel, for example? Consider the inflation rate. What income can you depend upon from Social Security, pensions, and other assets that generate income? This can be a little tricky and of course involves some speculation. That is why it is useful for your financial planner or CPA to "run the numbers." Just as businesses prepare pro forma projections, you need to develop different scenarios regarding your financial needs. The key is to be realistic and conservative. Most people don't have a clue what they need to retire.

3. How are you going to get there? Your journey to financial independence involves two strategies: a savings strategy

Financial Plan

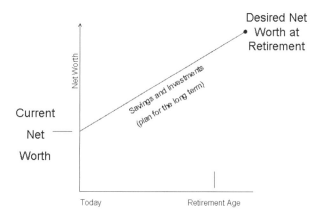

and an investment strategy. A savings strategy is deciding how much of your income you can save or how much spending you can defer. As illustrated later in this chapter, there are tremendous advantages to a Top-Down approach over the Bottom-Up approach. The investment strategy involves maximizing the return on your investments over that period of time. Your investment advisor can help you select a diversified portfolio that reflects your tolerance for risk. Assume a reasonable rate of return for your investments when estimating the results of your investment strategy. Naturally, your financial advisor can be of tremendous assistance in getting you there.

Saving. There are many products to help you save and reach your retirement. Tax-favored programs include a Rollover IRA, Traditional IRA, Roth IRA, Simplified Employee Pension (SEP) Program, and 401(k) plan.

- Rollover IRA. Distribution of assets from an employee-sponsored plan or another IRA into a Traditional IRA.
- Traditional IRA. Individual retirement plan that permits yearly contributions. Earnings grow tax deferred, and amounts withdrawn are taxed as ordinary income.
- Roth IRA. Individual retirement plan that permits nondeductible yearly contributions. Earnings grow tax deferred, and qualified distributions are tax free.
- Simplified Employee Pension (SEP). Economical tax-favored retirement program for self-employed individuals and small business owners.
- 401(k). Tax-favored retirement program sponsored by an employer.

By taking money directly from your salary, the above vehicles can be of tremendous help in saving. Generally, you want to save the maximum possible in these programs. Still, you need to prepare a budget. If you get anything out of this book, particularly this chapter, that is to establish a Top-Down Budget. As mentioned earlier, the savings rate of the baby-boomer generation in particular is dismal. In setting up your budget, remember that the first person you need to pay is yourself.

A budget can help you tremendously in your savings plan. Without a budget, it is simply too easy to spend money.

Remember that you are just one little consumer trying to hold on to your dollars in the face of all those producers of goods of all shapes and sizes, who constantly bombard you with ads to separate you from your money. A budget can empower you to just say no. A budget separates fixed items, such as mortgages and utilities, from discretionary costs, such as clothing and recreation.

If you are paid as an employee, you could start your budget with your net income. If you are paid as an independent contractor, budgeting is a little bit more difficult and you must withdraw taxes that you are going to later pay. Often it is helpful to put this in a separate account so that you are not tempted to touch the money. Getting behind on your taxes, just like getting behind on your credit cards, can lead to big problems quickly. The next step is to list all of your expenses. This would include your mortgage, utilities, car insurance, telephone, groceries, and all other major expenses. Then you want to set up a budget for items such as clothing, household expenses, and home repairs. Don't forget to include money for entertainment, dining, recreation, travel, and cleaning. Much of this latter category is discretionary spending, and you could exercise some discipline there in order to maximize savings. How much more could you save by dining out once a week instead of twice? In *The Automatic Millionaire*, the author calculated the cumulative effect of skipping a daily $3.50 cup of coffee at Starbucks. It is amazing how much you can save when you cut the "extras" from your budget. The key is not to compulsively track every nickel you spend but increase your savings rate as well as your enjoyment of what you do spend, because you can "budget" for it.

One advantage of a budget, like any set of goals, is that it makes you accountable. The budget helps you keep perspective and makes you less susceptible to impulse buying, since you have to live within that budget. You begin to see your finances in a big picture and understand where your money is going. Internet banking has allowed much readier access to your information, which can be downloaded into a financial software program. This also applies to your debit card. As in so many areas of your life, the key to tuning up your finances is to get a handle on them. Once you do that, they are much easier to manage.

Top-Down Budget
(vs. Traditional Bottom-Up Approach)

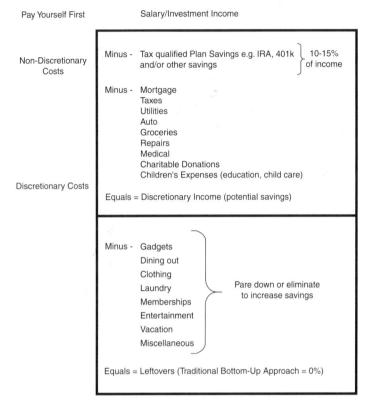

Pay Yourself First — Salary/Investment Income

Non-Discretionary Costs

Minus - Tax qualified Plan Savings e.g. IRA, 401k and/or other savings } 10-15% of income

Minus - Mortgage
Taxes
Utilities
Auto
Groceries
Repairs
Medical
Charitable Donations
Children's Expenses (education, child care)

Discretionary Costs

Equals = Discretionary Income (potential savings)

Minus - Gadgets
Dining out
Clothing
Laundry
Memberships
Entertainment
Vacation
Miscellaneous } Pare down or eliminate to increase savings

Equals = Leftovers (Traditional Bottom-Up Approach = 0%)

At a recent seminar, an economist stated that the American savings rate had in fact plunged to 0 percent, and people were instead living off of home-equity loans and recent gains in the stock market. You would think people might have learned something from the technology bubble. Instead, they are now being lured by the real-estate bubble.

Investment. Although this book does not purport to be an investment-strategy book, many books that claim to be actually are not. The truth is that even some of the best analysts on Wall Street are often wrong. Many people can predict the market in a broad sense looking at economic cycles. But predicting the performance of a single company in the short term is very difficult. Certain financial indicators affect the market, but numerous psychological and macro-economic factors may not be figured in. Consequently, it is difficult to predict stock prices on a short-term basis. However, on a long-term basis, the odds are much better for you, since stocks (like the economy) are cyclical. That's why you want to have diversified funds—that is, not overcommitted to a particular sector.

The next factor is market timing. Since it is very difficult to time the market, you are much better off making periodic investments as opposed to all at once. Therefore, a good investment strategy is to invest periodically into various mutual funds with a diversified portfolio that is tailored to your risk-return ratio, thereby assuring that you have a balanced portfolio. Many mutual funds (like defined contribution plans) will do a direct debit from your account, and that is one way to be sure that you are constantly investing in there. You will be surprised how quickly it can accumulate, from both appreciaton and the saving activity. By investing on a periodic basis, you can ensure that you are paying yourself first, as well as constant dollar averaging your investment.

Investing for the Long-term Perspective

> Endure and save yourself for happier times.
>
> —Virgil

As discussed earlier, steady investing over the long term produces the best results. A common mistake is investing for the short term instead of the long term. Too many try for this "quick" kill. However, perspective in your investment strategy requires many of the lessons we discussed earlier, including constant dollar averaging in a long-term investment strategy that is based on your tolerance for risk. This strategy should be adjusted for risk and return periodically according to your age. As discussed earlier, constant dollar averaging helps you avoid the highs and lows of the market. That was the entire premise of *The Automatic Millionaire.* We have also discussed several retirement vehicles to help with a long-run perspective, and Congress is always enacting more. The key is to diversify your portfolio and think long term. If you constantly make decisions based upon short-term results, you're doomed to have a less than average investment portfolio.

Incidentally, securities are not the only way to invest. In the book entitled *Rich Dad, Poor Dad,* which incidentally is an excellent investment book, the authors provide advice on becoming a level-one investor, someone who invests in income property and real estate as opposed to simply stock and brokerage accounts. Over the long term, you might want to think about real estate. If you don't like the upkeep of rental property, consider buying raw land.

Maintaining a long-term perspective about investing also involves protecting your money from taxes. Tax planning should be part of your financial independence strategy. Note that if you are trading an account, it makes more sense to do it in a tax-advantage account. If you are buying and selling real estate, there are sections under the Internal Revenue Code that allow tax exchanges. Tax planning is an important aspect of your investment strategy.

A long-term perspective not only addresses your financial independence but also ensures that all of your risks are covered. Do you have adequate insurance? Do you have disability insurance? What would happen in the event of extended illness or injury? These are all important issues that a good financial plan needs to address.

Avoid short-term risks and short-term rewards that many tend to brag about during boom periods. A long-term perspective will produce financial independence.

Financial Perseverance

> Money is a lot like the sixth sense without which you cannot make complete use of the other five.
> —W. Somerset Maugham, *Of Human Bondage*

As with everything else, one has to persevere in order to be successful. This is very important in the quest for financial independence. Financial independence is much like the story of the tortoise and hare. As we discussed earlier, the average millionaires in the United States are people who accumulated money slowly, not quickly. They generally owned their own businesses and accumulated and saved over a lifetime. They simply lived beneath their means and became millionaires through a careful and disciplined approach. That is why perseverance is so important. Set up a budget, savings strategy, and investment strategy, and stick to it.

The problem with many of the boomers is that they grew up

in the post-World War II years, during a time of unparalleled prosperity in the United States. Parts of Europe and Asia had been leveled by the war, and the United States had the capacity to produce the goods to rebuild them. When I was graduating from law school, the buzz was not about saving and investing for the long term but consuming in the short term. People were buying extravagant sports cars and homes instead of living modestly during the short term. One has to think constantly about the impact tomorrow of savings and investment decisions today. Most of all, day-to-day perseverance in long-term investing leads to financial independence. And remember that a penny saved is a penny earned.

CHAPTER 13

Career Tune-Up

Work perseveringly; work can be made into a pleasure,
and alone is profitable to man, to his city, to his country.
—Louis Pasteur

Become Passionate About Your Career

Life is just simply too short to remain trapped in a career that doesn't excite and challenge you. Many have become resigned to their career fate while the wondering in their hearts, "Is that all there is?" They feel trapped but worry that it's too late to do anything besides cling to the status quo. Although a career change might sound enticing, it is for younger people without bills to pay, mortgages to service, children to educate, and looming retirements to fund. Midlife is the time to hunker down, play defense, and simply try to hold on to your job. Did you know that there are more heart attacks on Monday than any other day? That's because too many of us are going to jobs that we can't stand.

But it doesn't have to be that way. Despite inevitable fluctuations in the economy and uncertainty in the world, we are still living in a period of tremendous opportunity. Small businesses are springing up daily to take advantage of unfulfilled needs and gaps in the marketplace, creating over 90 percent of the new jobs in the economy. I have written two books about entrepreneurship and have counseled and taught many entrepreneurs. In my experience, the essence of career passion is embodied by the entrepreneur. The term itself is derived from the French *entreprende,* to undertake. Passion and entrepreneurship are closely related because most entrepreneurs are driven by a career that they love and with which they are consumed, as opposed to just making money.

It is never too late to create a career that you love, one that you are truly passionate about. This does not necessarily mean you should quit your job to open your own business tomorrow, although it might. Entrepreneurship is risky, challenging, and rigorous and is certainly not for everyone. But you don't necessarily have to go out on your own to pursue a career that you love. Instead, tuning up your career requires that you be completely honest with yourself about your calling and then have the courage to follow through. The wife of a friend of mine left the corporate world at midlife for nursing school. She had urged her daughters to pursue a profession of helping people. When they did not show an interest, she did. She characterized the corporate world as "soulless" and began nursing school just before her fiftieth birthday. At first, she worried about looking ridiculous while attending school with students her daughters' age. But she found that she fit in just fine. Now she could not be happier with her decision.

Sometimes a career change is not always necessary. Adopting an entrepreneurial mindset can inject passion into your current job. Noted motivational author Brian Tracy points out that everyone is the president of their own "Personal Services Corporation." In other words, we are all providing services in one form or another with our work. Although we might be employed by someone else, the quantity and quality of the services we provide are completely within our control. We can view ourselves as bureaucrats, and do just what we need to get by, or as an entrepreneurs, constantly seeking to provide better solutions to our employers.

So keep abreast of the activity in your industry. Read all the annual reports of competitors. Learn the trends in your industry. Take the time to increase your own value. So if you're relatively happy where you are, your career tune-up plan is pretty simple: spend at least one hour a day educating yourself to become better at your job.

Passion often separates entrepreneurial employees from the others. Passionate employees think like entrepreneurs, scouring the landscape for new markets and opportunities and creating value for their employer. Average employees simply do their job and collect a paycheck. If you find yourself in a career or organization that does not challenge you to behave like an entrepreneur and go beyond your job description, then it might be time to reassess and find a new career you can become passionate about.

Work will always be work. Given a choice, most of us would

probably prefer our leisure time. But if you are feeling a little jaded in your career, it sometimes helps to take a fresh look at it and find a way to recover your passion. In my case, I was able to tune up my legal career by recovering my passion for law. I realized that I enjoyed working with entrepreneurs and helping businesses thrive. As long as I was in a fast-paced, productive business environment, I flourished. I became listless and unhappy when I was mired in more mundane legal work. That is why I switched from a private general practice to an in-house position with a dynamic, young company.

It's not always easy to recover passion for your present career. If you have always pictured yourself engaged in some other career or activity, then it might be time to consider making a change. I know firsthand how difficult changing careers at midstream can be. Such a career about-face often requires considerable courage and can pose significant hardships. After spending many years mastering one profession, leaving it behind can feel frightening and wasteful at the same time.

Boomers in particular have been conditioned to think that career passion should be subordinate to security. The career model that was instilled was to go to school, get a job with a good company, work hard, and place your entire career in the hands of the company. Ignore any career passion and accept transfers and new assignments willingly while giving the company your complete loyalty. In exchange for this loyalty and service, the employees were given lifetime employment, medical benefits, security for their family, and, of course, the proverbial gold watch. This was known as the social contract between corporate America and the workforce.

Under this paradigm, individual career decisions were not entirely within a person's control. Although they could express preferences, employees usually performed the particular job and in the particular city that their company wanted them to. Believe it or not, when I attended business school, there were no courses in entrepreneurship. You simply learned certain theoretical business tools, which would be later shaped by your employer. Today, entrepreneurship courses are the most popular at the university. If any of my classmates had told me back in the 1980s that they were going to start their own business, I would have figured that their grades were not good enough for them to land a decent job.

Of course, this social contract between corporate American and the workforce began to change dramatically in the 1980s. The manufacturing sector was the first area to be affected. As this sector was forced to retool to compete with revitalized foreign competitors, blue-collar jobs began to disappear. Domestic factories were shut down due to cheaper imports and cheaper labor costs overseas. The white-collar workforce was generally spared until the 1990s, when a competitive global marketplace forced the restructuring of the traditional American corporation. Suddenly, white-collar jobs began to vanish also, with the sometimes carnage euphemistically referred to as "reengineering." The social contract between corporate employers and employees had been broken. Some employees who had given their whole careers to one company were rewarded with pink slips during the prime of their working years. My own employer morphed almost overnight from a model of benevolence that could not do enough for its employees to a relentless cost-cutting machine.

This abrupt change in workforce attitudes and practices has both positive and negative implications. Since there is no longer any security in the workforce, why not pursue a career that you enjoy and that stirs your passion? Take the initiative to create your own career plan. Take an aggressive stance in advancing and reshaping your own career rather than depending on your employer to do so.

Many boomers find themselves in the position of receiving early retirement or severance packages in midcareer. This can be a bit disconcerting to someone, including myself, who was used to the security and structure of an employer. Suddenly Monday rolls around, and there's no place to "go." Although this could initially seem like a "bad break," resolve to bounce back in a career that you love. This could be your chance to finally pursue a career that you've always dreamed about.

Early retirement can be a vulnerable time, and it is important to think clearly. Don't rush to accept any job or go out and invest in the first "business opportunity" that comes your way. For example, realize that owning a franchise can sometimes be nothing more than buying a job. Before you invest money in a franchise, thoroughly investigate it.

A good friend of mine refused a company transfer in his

fifties and decided to start his own business, which was making uniforms and custom apparel for businesses. He investigated and found that such clothing was often inferior and he could provide superior customized clothing at competitive prices. His business skyrocketed and he plowed the resources back into his company, completely computerizing his operations. Today he seems happier than ever, almost amazed at his own success. But it only occurred when he had the courage to take his career into his own hands.

Stories abound about people who created very successful careers at midlife. For every child prodigy, there are hundreds of people who soared at midcareer. We already examined the remarkable career of Ray Kroc, the founder of McDonald's. Victor Kiam made a modest living until he read an article in *Business Week* about a razor manufacturer being put up for sale. Although Kiam didn't have much money, he was able to scrape together the resources to buy Remington. His book entitled *Going for It* details his entrepreneurial vision and how an ordinary person can do very well, well enough to afford to buy the New England Patriots. Most of us would be happy succeeding on a much smaller scale. You don't need to be trapped in a career rut. New information, new ideas, and, most importantly, a belief in yourself can propel your career.

Nearly 80 percent of the wealth in this country is created by entrepreneurs, people who are willing to step out of their comfort zones and take risks with their careers. Those who are successful take educated financial risks and are not afraid to invest in themselves, their careers, and their professional practices. They focus on success instead of failure. The best way to become passionate about your career is to choose a career path that you believe fulfills your unique purpose.

Uncovering Your Unique Career Purpose

> Believe in yourself! Have faith in your abilities. Without a humble but reasonable confidence in your own powers you cannot be successful or happy.
>
> —Norman Vincent Peale

Midlife can be a perfect time to reflect upon your career purpose. Be honest with yourself. Perhaps you've always wanted to do something else, like the lawyer-turned-doctor I wrote of earlier. Although he buried his head in law books during the day, his mind was filled with images of himself in a white coat. What work clothes do you imagine yourself in?

By midlife, you have the advantage of work and life experience and are more aware of the activities or industries that suit you. Your career purpose might be fulfilled by switching jobs in one industry or switching industries but with the same job.

Finding your career purpose may involve discovering what is known as your career "niche." Just as businesses search for that segment of the market where they outshine their competitors and offer the most value to consumers, individuals can benefit from finding their own niche, which takes the best advantage of their unique talents and where they can offer the highest value. Being paid well for something you enjoy and excel at can significantly enhance your career. Your niche could be that part of the market or career that you have mastered. A career niche can help you focus more accurately on your purpose and lead to greater financial rewards.

Another way to view a career niche is as one's career specialty. The specialists in particular professions are usually the highest paid. For example, specialists in such areas as law, medicine, and accounting are usually paid better than generalists, and they also seem to enjoy their work more. For example, professions like law can be quite broad and most general practitioners I know don't seem to particularly enjoy the practice. However, those who specialize seem much happier. They are doing something that they really like as opposed to whatever walks in the door, and they have genuine passion for their careers. It never ceases to amaze me how excited some of my contemporaries become talking about something as mundane as tax law. They enjoy going to the conferences, reading the journals, discovering the different ideas, and always seeking better ways to offer their services.

Sometimes you can create your own niche from different careers, contacts, and opportunities. My late stepfather found his career niche in midlife after going through a difficult divorce. Not only did his former wife crush his heart, but she hired a particularly aggressive divorce specialist to go after his bank account. Rather than lament this bad fortune, my stepfather resolved to rebuild himself emotionally and financially.

Part of this rebuilding process involved discovering his career niche. My stepfather worked as a hairdresser. Later, he supplemented his income by selling real estate on the weekends. However, it was the unlikely combination of hairdressing and real estate where he finally flourished. His salon was located on the first floor of a pricey high-rise apartment building on exclusive St. Charles Avenue in Uptown New Orleans. Since my stepfather was skilled and personable, many of the residents were his clients. A few years later, when the apartment building was converted to condominiums, he found himself on the ground floor of a significant market opportunity in the resales of the condominium units. His salon clients who knew he was in real estate listed their properties with him for sale. Word began to spread, and those looking to buy in the complex would use him also, because his salon contacts provided the scoop of who might be planning to move but whose property had not yet hit the marketplace. Pretty soon he was doing the bulk of his real-estate work in one building instead of running all over the city.

What career niche might by lying under your nose? In addition to your specialized knowledge, your contacts and chutzpah to follow through contribute to creating your niche.

In his book *What Color Is Your Parachute?* author Richard Nelson Bolles outlines a series of tests to help determine your career path. The key is to match your unique abilities with a market niche. A good match can make you very happy as well as successful. Your career niche is closely related to your uniqueness. Everyone has unique talents. Everyone also has certain career dreams and aspirations, however fleeting they may be. But sometimes others, including—unfortunately—our parents and friends, discourage us from pursuing our dreams. Often, our inner voice is the loudest critic of all. It can stifle our aspirations so that we never act upon them. Graveyards are full of buried dreams.

A career niche can be created by looking for problems and producing solutions. There are always opportunities or gaps in the marketplace where someone with superior knowledge can outshine competitors. My stepfather simply became an authority on that particular building. He had the most knowledge, information, and contacts about the markets and made the best of them. It is not necessarily the revolutionary ideas that create the career niche. Rather, it is the willingness to understand the market and being proactive enough to simply get out there and "do it."

We often cross paths with exciting opportunities in our day-to-day lives. Such opportunities could contribute to our purpose of creating a viable business. Good ideas are plentiful but can die on the vine if you do not take the initiative and execute them. How many times have you seen a best-selling product and then mumbled to yourself, "I could have thought of that"? The truth is that you could have. It is not that people lack creativity; they don't give themselves enough credit for having it.

The book *The Power Years,* by Ken Dychtwald, recommends these steps in choosing a career niche.

1. Get in a relaxed place, preferably alone or in a tranquil setting. Take the time to give serious thought to what you might want to do.
2. Clear your mind. For a moment, forget about everything you think you should do. Reflect on all of your previous jobs (including volunteer ones) and consider what you liked about each. Were any ambitions of your youth derailed by practical considerations?
3. Remember that there are no rules; just let your ideas flow.
4. Ask yourself the following questions:
   a. If I could do anything in the world, what would it be?
   b. What career would I choose if there was no risk of failure?
   c. How could I make this a viable business?
5. Identify how you spend your discretionary income. This can help you recognize your priorities.
6. Look for opportunities in fields that have labor shortages and that are open to older workers.
7. Go back to school for additional training and credentials.

For those who are serious about starting a business, the best place to begin is to prepare a business plan. Although the failure prospects for a new business can be intimidating, my experience is that those who prepare a business plan have a better than average chance of succeeding. A turnaround specialist that I know has never had to rescue a client who had a good business plan. The good news is that you can prepare a business plan at any time, and the mere fact that you write one doesn't obligate or bind you in any way.

Preparing a business plan can be a time-consuming and exacting process. However, like the proverbial weightlifter, you can't get the gain without the pain. The discipline of sitting down and working through your plan really forces you to confront some of the tough questions about the prospective business. Is there an adequate market? How much money will I need to get started? How will I handle the competition? The business plan leads you through the issues and strategies of successfully running your business. Although the task might appear overwhelming at first, remember that the key to accomplishing any large job is to break it up into separate pieces. Also, the Small Business Administration has Small Business Development Centers (affiliated with many area universities), which can furnish resources to assist in preparing your business plan.

Elements of a Business Plan

Executive Summary (Statement of Purpose). The purpose of the executive summary is to provide an overview of the business, which would include the product or service that you offer and the market that you serve. In other words, the executive summary describes your vision for the business and your strategy for competing in the market.

Management and Organization. The management and organization section of the business plan is the portion where you would discuss the management team, their backgrounds, and the legal form of your business. Although you may not have an executive management team, note that the financial, marketing, and legal functions all need to be fulfilled. In some of these areas, you might need outside help, particularly the financial area.

Description of the Product/Service. This part of the plan contains a detailed description of the purpose of your product or service. The key is to emphasize the *unique* features of your product or service. Elaborate on the benefits of your goods and services from your customers' perspective. You could also mention the history of the product or service and any spin-off or related products or services. This description would also include a profile of the industry that you will be operating in. The industry profile consists of the size of your market, the type of market, and your growth potential. Next, you would make a competitive analysis of similar products and services. It is useful to prepare a competitive matrix profile, in which you compare yourself with your competitors in areas such as price, quality, selection, additional services, and facilities or locations and distinguish your product from theirs.

Marketing Plan. The marketing plan begins with a profile of your customer. Who is your customer? What is your target market? The key element of a successful marketing plan is knowing your customers—their likes, dislikes, expectations. By identifying these factors, you can develop a marketing strategy that will allow you to address their needs. The goal is to target your market by identifying customers by their age, sex, income/educational level, and residence. Successful businesses carefully select one or more target markets for their marketing efforts.

The marketing portion of the plan would address the marketing mix (product, place, price) and the promotional strategies used to reach the target market. Your product or service is naturally one of the most important parts of the marketing mix, and your marketing plan needs to focus on those unique aspects for promotion to your target market. Promotional techniques, such as print and Internet advertising, media, and public relations, need to be used in a manner that conveys your message. Other important parts of your marketing mix are your pricing and distribution strategies.

Financial Data. The necessary financial data includes the initial capital requirements, which are the resources needed to get a business up and running. Next would be the projection of operating results. This involves the accounting tools of the startup budget, pro forma cash-flow statements, and balance sheets. The financial data is the glue that holds the rest of the plan together. If you don't have a financial background, it is useful to have a CPA or someone at a Small Business Development Center help you prepare your financial projections.

Appendices. The appendices of your business plan would contain such items as product literature, articles about the business, your résumé, relevant research, and anything else that you feel is pertinent to the business.

Although drawing up a business plan appears to be tedious at first, the best way to prepare one is to just get started. Go to your computer and type the cover page and table of contents. On the contents page, list all of the parts of the business plan: executive summary (statement of purpose), management and organization, description of the product/service, marketing plan, financial data, and appendices. Then, type these same parts at the top of separate pages. Congratulations! Now you've got the outline of your business plan.

I wanted to offer a few final thoughts on self-employment. Although it is true that some people are more temperamentally suited for entrepreneurship than others, don't immediately count yourself out. The biggest hurdle is to change your *belief* about self-employment. For the first-time entrepreneur, who might have spent much of their career working in a corporation, being on their own is a strange and frightening prospect. These are normal feelings for anyone who trades in a steady paycheck for something much less certain.

We can always focus on the risks of self-employment. Although the majority of startups fail in the first five years, such business failure can be attributed to the lack of knowledge in key business areas, such as finance, accounting, management, and law. With proper education and planning, you can actually turn the success ratio in your favor.

That is why it is so important to empower yourself before starting your business, so that you have confidence in your ability and resources. As we have discussed, such confidence can be derived from inner faith, past success, and the realization that many others have succeeded in business.

Another key to successful self-employment is being proactive. New ideas have to be implemented quickly. Learn to take action *today*, not tomorrow.

Being proactive involves the ability to synthesize information and make decisions. Entrepreneurs often make dozens of decisions in a single day. Therefore, they must be comfortable with their decision-making process.

I read a recent article in *Business Week* concerning people changing careers at midlife. A Merrill Lynch retirement survey of more than three thousand boomers reported that 83 percent intended to keep working and 56 percent of them hoped to do so in a new profession. One sixty-seven-year-old woman wanted a career change after running a human-resources company in Manhattan for twenty-five years. She eventually became certified as a personal trainer. A fifty-six-year-old man, who worked three decades as a civil litigator in San Francisco, decided to change careers and become a minister. He completed a three-year graduate seminary program at Graduate Theological Union in Berkeley. A CEO of a hair-products company became CEO of Girls, Inc., a national nonprofit dedicated to helping girls. A retired rheumatologist sold his medical practice and opened an ice-cream shop. And the list went on. All of these people empowered themselves at midlife or beyond to pursue their newfound purposes.

Empowering Your Career

> If you don't get a kick out of the job you are doing, you'd better hunt another one.
>
> —Samuel Vaucloin

The quickest way to empower your career is to concentrate on creating more value for your customers and/or employer. Two ways to create value are (1) developing a specialized skill, knowledge, methodology, or product, and/or (2) creating market appeal and bringing in customers.

Consider some of the wealthiest individuals, whose ranks include star athletes and entertainers. They have been able to combine both a specialized skill with market appeal. Professional athletes such as Tiger Woods and Michael Jordan not only commanded high compensation but also significant endorsement fees, because their exceptional skills made them hot market commodities. Bill Gates is another example of someone who was able to combine a specialized product—in his case, the operating software for the new personal computer—with market appeal. Gates' vision and tenacity allowed him to dominate the computer software market and made him the world's richest person.

I know that the vast majority of us are not superstar athletes, entertainers, or chairmen of one of the world's most valuable companies. Still, a specialized skill or market appeal can propel our career, while the combination of both can be especially effective. Let me explain.

Many of the higher-paid professions are those requiring specialized skills—neurosurgery, information technology, and intellectual property protection, for example. By increasing your knowledge of your industry or company, you can offer more value to your employer. Consequently, the first way to empower your career is increase your level of skill and knowledge. The more you know, the more value you can create. Lawyers, musicians, athletes, and marketing professionals can command extremely high compensation when they are perceived to be the best in their professions. Those at the very top of their profession are often paid as much as five to ten times more than their contemporaries, even though they are not five to ten times better. People are always willing to pay top dollar for the "best." Consider professional baseball. A baseball player who consistently hits over .300 can be paid many millions, while someone who hits .225 will be paid considerably less. It's hard to understand why the higher-paid athlete is perceived as so much more valuable than the lower-paid counterpart, when the difference in performance is not that great. But when you focus on excelling at your profession, such incremental improvements in skill can command considerably higher compensation.

Consequently, seize every opportunity to become better at what you do. All the top performers are constantly honing their skills. Attend seminars. Read books. Listen to CDs. Talk to high performers in your field. They have worked hard to rise to the top. The little advantages can accumulate and add up to big returns. As mentioned before, sometimes spending just one hour a day to improve your career can yield large dividends.

The next way to empower your career is through enhancing your marketing ability and knowledge, particularly if marketing is not your expertise. Our information-savvy society has created a more demanding consumer. During the manufacturing age, consumers were captives of the large manufacturers. The height of industrial arrogance was summarized in Henry Ford's remark about his Model-T—his customers could have any color car they wanted so long as it was black. Today, the consumer is in the driver's seat, and the competition for their business is intense. If you don't satisfy them, then somebody else will. The most successful professionals are proficient at marketing. It is no accident that top salespeople are paid as well as the most skilled physicians. After all, they bring customers in the door, and you can't have a business without customers. In addition, it is often not what you know but also who you know. Therefore, go the extra mile to meet and develop contacts. Networking is an important form of marketing. No matter what you do, there is always value in knowing the right people. In fact, contacts can literally make or break your career. It never ceases to amaze me how the right contacts have helped me at critical times. That is why it is important to adopt an aggressive marketing attitude. Every person you meet is a potential client and customer for your business. Go the extra mile to become active, involved, and well known in your community or profession. This can serve to greatly increase your value and assist your career.

Business is all about people and understanding the needs of the marketplace. Despite our highly technical world, with its e-mail, faxes, and remote offices, people are still very much social creatures. They tend to do business with people they like. Therefore, take the time to build up your database of contacts and leads to increase your value and further tune up your career. Some choose technical professions simply because they don't like dealing with people. However, why lock yourself away, often working for somebody else, while the ones who soar have combined their technical skills with marketing activities?

Value can be an elusive concept. In the free market in which we live, we are compensated for the value that we create. This value can be as much *perceived* as actual. If you are perceived to provide value, then someone will pay for your product or service. Do you ever wonder why people line up at Starbucks to pay three and four dollars for coffee that might cost Starbucks less than fifty cents to produce? I have seen teenagers pay as much for coffee and a Danish at Starbucks as I pay for lunch. But Starbucks provides the experience that people are more than willing to pay for. Starbucks provides "perceived" value.

If you create value for either your company or your customers, find a way to let the right people know. Don't be shy about requesting compensation for creating value or charging for the value you create. Why do you think that investment bankers are so well compensated? They are perceived to provide value in the form of financial resources for their clients. I once heard popular televangelist Joyce Meyer speak in New Orleans. In the middle of her presentation, she made a direct appeal for donations, which was based upon her value creation. She asked how many in the packed arena watched her show. Of course, everyone's hands went up. She then asked how many benefited from the show. All the hands went up again. Then she closed with the phrase, "If you're getting a benefit at McDonald's, you don't pay Burger King." Her logic impressed the audience, and the donations flowed in.

Empowering your career involves learning how to create value. Bureaucratic organizations can create a disconnect between value creation and actual skill. What can you do to create value? Find new markets? Make the organization run more effectively? Make suggestions to improve the bottom line? Create new products? Help raise capital? The list is endless if you're willing to do some research and think outside of the box.

A final thought on career empowerment: many of us are held back in our careers by the things we simply don't like to do. We find it much easier to plow through meaningless paperwork or answer e-mails than to focus on important activities, such as large projects that will increase our value to our employers. You might know that you should be prospecting for larger accounts, but you spend time with smaller accounts that you're more comfortable with. You might show up at the office all charged up for a productive day but allow yourself to be sidetracked by meaningless distractions. Those who have succeeded have overcome this tendency to procrastinate and have empowered themselves. They focused their energy on the important activities until they were finished and were not afraid to take reasonable and necessary risks. This seems quite simple but can be difficult to carry out. However, this type of empowerment can greatly assist in advancing your career.

Mapping Out Your Career Plan

Formulate and stamp indelibly on your mind a mental picture of yourself as succeeding. Hold this picture tenaciously. Never permit it to fade. Your mind will seek to develop the picture.

—Norman Vincent Peale

To map out your career plan, you'll need to make the following assessments.

1. Decide whether or not you are happy in your current career. Remember that sometimes, by changing your industry or job, you can employ existing skills and refine your career into one you are passionate about.
2. If you are happy in your career, tune up by creating more value and increasing your technical and marketing skills.
3. Create a business plan in which you seek to understand the market and industry and work to create more value in your occupation. Do the necessary market research; in other words, research the industry, competition, and your customer. Position yourself to add more value to your job.
4. If you're not happy in your career, perhaps consult with a career counselor. Or pay attention to that little voice inside and investigate potential career changes. This could culminate in a plan to change careers and even start your own business. We discussed earlier the necessity of a business plan in starting a business.
5. In many cases, a career change will necessitate additional education. We have already discussed the examples of the lawyer turned doctor, lawyer turned minister, and human-resources executive turned personal fitness trainer. All sought the necessary education to change careers.

If you decide that a changing your career path is advisable, your tune-up plan could be a bit more involved. The lawyer turned doctor made an about-face in order to wear the white coat. However, his deep-seated desire simply would not go away. If you are constantly thinking about another career, then you need to take some due diligence and investigate it. I knew a laid-off aerospace engineer who wanted to open his own restaurant, or at least he thought he did. Since he knew nothing about the field, he wrote five letters requesting an internship. Three responded and he spent several weeks at a restaurant out of state learning the tricks of the trade, but more importantly "feeling" what it was like to run a restaurant. The grass always looks greener from the outside, and if you are seriously thinking about changing professions, it might be wise to spend some time in that profession before making the leap. This man started a restaurant called The Broken Egg, which serves breakfast and lunch in Mandeville, Louisiana. It was a big hit. Soon he began franchising in the Southeast and is doing very well.

The more hands-on experience you can obtain in a prospective career, the better off you will be. Don't just look for a new career that seems like the "thing" to do. Often a career area that is hot one day can turn cold the next. Also be wary of get-rich-quick schemes. There is an entire industry built around duping people who are not happy with their current jobs into doing something such as setting up 900 numbers, various Internet and network marketing ventures, and other schemes that in most cases enrich the founders but leave their "students" considerably less wealthy and searching for the next easy scheme. Beware of anything that claims you can become financially independent working ten hours per week. Instead take responsible steps to determine a new career direction. Take the time to investigate and, even as my friend did, experience a new career. Talk to friends and associates, but filter their advice. Many will urge the safest path, while others have no idea what they're talking about. There are also unfortunately some people who really don't want you to succeed. Tap a few trusted sources for information.

While you might share your idea for a new business with others, don't be discouraged by their reactions. A complete discussion on starting a new business can be found in my earlier book entitled *Break the Curve: The Entrepreneur's Blueprint for Small Business Success.* Taking the idea for a new business venture and turning it into reality requires research and careful preparation of a business plan. In my opinion, if everyone tells you that your business is a good idea, then you have a problem. Be prepared to do the necessary work to turn your idea or dream into a reality. My clients who have started businesses have widely varying backgrounds of education, experience, and resources. Many of their ideas seemed preposterous at first. But even college students have developed blueprints for viable businesses after just a few weeks of class. They are generally in their final spring semester, and it never ceases to amaze me how these often less than serious young people, with already one foot out the door of the university, can team up and develop viable business plans, possibly over drinks at an area pub.

Imagine what you can do with your experience if you really focus. Everyone has a creative potential, but few actually believe in it, and even fewer actually exercise it. We all have been given certain gifts and talents that can be parlayed into successful careers. Such talents don't necessarily have to be those of a star athlete or technology wizard. Consider the story of Debbie Fields, the founder of Mrs. Fields cookies. As a young housewife in Palo Alto, she found herself intimidated by those around her with degrees and careers. When she had the urge to start a business in her early twenties, she inventoried her own talents. The one that stood out was her ability to bake cookies. She was the youngest of several daughters, and while growing up, each of them participated in preparing some aspect of the family meal. As the caboose in her household, Debbie specialized in desserts. She took great care to use fresh, homemade ingredients to bake her cookies. So a cookie shop was the logical business for her to start. She was finally able to secure a bank loan for her first cookie shop. The night before her shop opened, she sat down with her husband and they figured out that she would have to sell $200 worth of cookies daily to break even. But by noon of her first day, she hadn't sold a single cookie. Yet instead of sitting back and waiting for the customers to come to her, she walked up and down the Palo Alto street offering her cookies to pedestrians. Many followed her back into the store and bought cookies. By the end of the first day, she had sold $200 worth, and the rest, of course, is history. This one store led to an international cookie empire that was sold for over $600 million.

In my experience, those who succeeded in their careers were able to leverage their contacts, knowledge, and ability, and they believed in themselves.

Maintaining a Career Perspective

The great secret of power is—save your force. If you want high pressure, you must choke off the waste.

—Henrik Ibsen

Consider your career from your own perspective as opposed to others' perspectives. When you are setting your career goals and asking yourself the tough questions, focus on the inside. It is so easy to become distracted or discouraged when we compare ourselves to others. Invariably, there are others whom we perceive as more successful than us. However, we have to plan our strategy from our own perspective. Forget about the others and concentrate on yourself. Someone will always do better than you, no matter what you do.

It is important to keep a long-term perspective with respect to your career. Too many people become impatient or easily discouraged. Career success depends on perseverance and sticking it out. Don't expect to invent the newest software program or hit television show overnight. It is often the little things that you do that lead up to larger accomplishments. While you should work on attracting larger clients, be sure not to shortchange your smaller ones. I had to make the transition in law from dealing with multinational corporations to ordinary people off the street. In restarting my law practice, I resolved to do the best I could with the people who were my clients at the time. I needed to be patient and keep perspective in building my business. Slowly, the smaller clients became larger clients, and then I was able to join one as their general counsel.

Have patience! History is full of people who tried and tried and only towards the end of their careers were they finally successful. Entertainment figures from Liberace to Metallica toiled for years before succeeding in their profession. I recently read a *Wall Street Journal* story on best-selling author James Patterson. Patterson has established a formidable publishing empire, with his income estimated at $25 million annually. Although he experienced some setbacks, he persisted in the marketing of his own books. He learned marketing as a copywriter for J. Walter Thompson. He struggled as a novelist for years and finally used his marketing background to shift his literary career into high gear. However, he did not depend solely on his publisher to market his books. He took matters into his own hands, even paying for his own television commercial after his publisher refused to do so. And he didn't reach real success until midlife.

Career Perseverance

> Give me a standing place and I will move the world. [Give me a lever long enough and I could move the world.]
>   —Archimedes

One common denominator in résumés of successful people is perseverance. It is rare for someone to succeed on their first attempt. The president of Atari told Steve Jobs, "You stink. Get your feet off my desk. And we're not going to buy any of your products." Of course, Jobs parlayed his Apple Computers into a worldwide success. And one skeptic asked Walt Disney, "Who in the world is going to buy a talking mouse?" We all know how that turned out.

Perseverance in your career is important. So many people have quit just as they were about to achieve success. Usually, the larger the endeavor, the more perseverance is required. Success in any field involves the ability to handle massive rejection and not give up. The best-selling series *Chicken Soup for the Soul* was rejected by thirty-seven publishers. It took over two years for the agent of best-selling author John Grisham to find a publisher for his first book, *A Time to Kill.* In fact, Grisham kept bugging his agent so much that the agent instructed him to quit calling and start a second book. It was actually this second book, *The Firm,* that propelled Grisham to literary superstardom. Had his first book been sold quickly, Grisham may never have written a second.

CHAPTER 14

Relationship Tune-Up

Your day breaks, your mind aches,
You find that all the words of kindness linger on
When she no longer needs you.
She wakes up, she makes up,
She takes her time and doesn't feel she has to hurry.
She no longer needs you.

And in her eyes you see nothing,
No sign of love behind the tears
Cried for no one,
A love that should have lasted years!
    —John Lennon and Paul McCartney, "For No One"

These immortal and haunting lyrics stand as a testament to today's failed relationships, generally due to neglect by one or both parties. Unfortunately, relationships take work, a lot of work, which includes constant communication, a willingness to compromise, and a deep commitment. A relationship cannot simply be placed on cruise control and be expected to hum along intact. I mistakenly believed otherwise, and it caused a lot of problems in my past relationships.

In fact, I even hesitate to provide any advice on relationships, because it has been such difficult area in my life. But on the flip side, if I can finally have a successful long-term relationship, then you can too.

Healthy romantic relationships are the basis of our society. The married couple forms the foundation of the family unit. Children who are reared in a stable loving home are generally much better adjusted than those who are raised in a less supportive environment. Still, relationships are a difficult area and can even be tricky for the experts. Consider that two of the leading books on relationships were written by authors who were formerly married to each other. John Gray wrote about the impact of gender differences on relationships in a best-selling book entitled *Men Are from Mars, Women Are from Venus.* His former wife, Barbara De Angelis, wrote the acclaimed book on evaluating a potential mate entitled *Are You the One for Me?* If two best-selling experts on relationships can't remain married to each other, that provides quite a challenge for the rest of us.

The high divorce rate in this country seemingly bears this out. As mentioned earlier, the divorce rate in this country remains over 50 percent, with the initial rise being driven by baby boomers. Prior to the advent of the boomers, couples were more likely to stick it out for better or worse. Today, there is considerable cynicism about marriage and commitment in general. In a book entitled *Why Can't I Fall in Love?* rabbi and counselor Shmuley Boteach points out that much of the current lack of commitment and love is due to fundamental shifts in society. In the generation that preceded baby boomers, the entire social structure was built around dating. People courted for a period of time and then they married, usually in their early twenties. There was tremendous anticipation for getting married and moving out of the house. Often, marriage was the ticket to physical intimacy. Instead of being thought of as confining, marriage was actually perceived as liberating.

Then came the sixties and the individual expression and permissiveness that accompanied the sexual revolution. Suddenly, free love was in vogue and people were not placing marriage before intimacy. There was less urgency to marry or remain married. As the seventies and eighties wore on, two-income households emerged as women began to enter the workforce. Women were no longer dependent on men for their financial security. Today, individuals tend to focus on individual career accomplishments at the expense of their dependence on others. Such dependence, often a critical factor in entering into or remaining in a marriage, is something that our society subtly frowns on. This aversion to being dependent on another can be a significant factor in preventing people from pairing up or staying together. You have to be willing to lose a bit of yourself to enjoy a successful relationship. In previous generations, people would change jobs, careers, houses, cities, all in the name of love. People today are less willing to compromise. But if you want success in your relationship, you have to be willing to compromise.

The irony is that the high divorce rate persists despite studies that show that married people are generally the happiest. Yet many continue to struggle with relationships and have difficulty finding and remaining in a committed relationship with a suitable life partner. Sometimes these problems stem from our approach to dating. Although you might wonder about the timeliness of a dating guide for those in midlife, I had many divorced and single friends, including myself, who needed to brush up on their approach to dating. If you are married, you can skip this section or perhaps pick up some pointers for your available friends.

Dating 101

The first step for those of us who are not married or in a committed relationship, but who would like to be, is to remove the cynicism from our lives. We have all been hurt in the past. I have been ditched, jettisoned, tossed, dumped more times than I can remember. However, in order to give ourselves the best chance to "fall in love," we have to brush aside the past and give romance a chance.

Next you need to examine what you are looking for. Too many of us are looking for perfection and, in some cases, a mirror image of ourselves. We have been brainwashed with the notion that there is some perfect person out there for us and we measure our prospects with arbitrary, lofty expectations. Instead, we need to be more tolerant of the differences in others and, in particular, less judgmental about their appearance. How many times do we cross off a potential suitor quickly on the basis of first physical impressions and don't take the time to get to know them? Although physical chemistry is necessary for a relationship to gel, be reasonable in setting the criteria.

The next bit of advice is to be proactive. I know how difficult it is being "out there." I hated singles bars just as much as everyone else does. Although dating can be intimidating, it can be fun if you let it and if you make the effort to meet others. In my opinion, the best way to meet someone is to try a little bit of everything. This includes online dating services, being fixed up by friends, going to different socials and mixers, and simply keeping your eyes open. Often the person you wish to meet is not conveniently introduced to you, so you have to find a way to meet them. This applies to women as well as men. Sometimes you have to be quick on your feet to initiate a conversation that doesn't appear as though you are trying to meet them (although both of you know otherwise). Also, don't be afraid to fix your friends up if you come across someone who would be suitable. I have had so many people tell me "I've got just the right person for you" and then they never do anything about it. Make the effort to help someone. It could change their lives. It can be hard out there, and anything you do to help someone is appreciated. Also, don't be shy in letting your friends know that you are interested in a relationship. It also doesn't hurt to have friends of the opposite sex, as they can help you meet others.

One of the techniques mentioned above that is generating interest and even results is dating over the Internet. Although some of my friends compare it to a digital meat market, the services are gaining in usage and popularity. A former secretary of mine, who was in her fifties, grew tired of the traditional dating scene after three failed marriages and many more failed relationships, particularly her last one with a noncommittal attorney. She had heard all the excuses about why someone could not get married and wanted to hear someone "pop the question." Her two daughters had completed college and moved out, and the family pet had gone on to dog heaven. Her Internet listing was brief and to the point: "Got rid of the kids and the dog and want to settle down with the right guy." She made it quite clear that she was very serious about settling down. Within a few months, she met someone from North Carolina, moved there, and got married.

All of the sites have fairly detailed profiles of their members, including age, interests, and requirements in a mate. The site e-harmony.com features a twenty-six-point profile that is used to ensure maximum compatibility. In the book *Date or Soul Mate? How to Know If Someone Is Worth Pursuing in Two Dates or Less,* Dr. Neil Clark Warren, the founder of e-harmony, goes into great detail about his compatibility system and its advantages over "traditional" dating. According to Dr. Warren, traditional dating emphasizes physical attractiveness over the compatibility factors. We tend to gravitate towards people to whom we are physically attracted and then work on compatibility later. Instead, we should focus upon those with whom we are compatible before even judging physical characteristics. This is consistent with Rabbi Boteach's recommendation that you give someone a chance even if there is no initial physical attraction.

So if you've not had much luck in dating lately, give the Internet a chance. I have a female friend who enjoys the convenience of Internet dating while she tries to balance life as a single working mother in her thirties. It's amazing what you learn about yourself during the Internet dating process and from the thought-provoking questions from other participating members. It's important to maintain an open mind. Although there may not be a connection at first, you just never know. A good example of this is an exchange of e-mails my friend had with an individual who originally sparked her interest but failed to maintain it, only to be introduced by a mutual friend a month later. They recognized each other from the Internet site and immediately hit it off. Had it not been for the arranged meeting, nothing would have materialized.

One question to consider, regardless of your methods of finding dates, is "what am I getting?" If you seem to be ending up with people who are already in relationships, who live in a different city, or who are abusive or self-absorbed, then you have to ask yourself whether or not there is a pattern with your relationships. How many people do you know (including maybe yourself) keep ending up in dead-end relationships? Reflect on the people whom you have dated in the past and determine if there is a pattern, or more accurately, a problem.

The next question to consider is "what can I do to change?" This involves changing both yourself and your choices. Decide to dust yourself off from previous failures and hurts and approach dating with a new perspective. I am not trying to defend the male population, but I really don't think that all guys are rats. Many of my female friends tell me that men have all the advantages in dating or that there are no good men left. Although in some parts of the country single men might have a slight numerical advantage, it certainly is not overwhelming. Some of your problems could stem from the fact you are not giving others a real chance. If you are not finding what you want, then you might want to relax your criteria a little bit. I am not saying that you settle, but at least give people a chance. Go out with someone for at least two dates, even if you strongly suspect in the first five minutes that they are probably not for you.

I have a good friend whose fiancée canceled their wedding. Although understandably devastated, he quickly rebounded, picking up the pieces of his broken heart and putting together a plan to find a wife, since he was ready to get married. Although terribly self-conscious about being both short and bald, he dated methodically (using some of the methods discussed above) and persisted despite considerable rejection along the way. But in the end, he found a woman who stole his heart and really loved him for who he was. Today he is happily married with a family. But he would have never ended up in this enviable state if he hadn't been so dedicated to dating and willing to handle rejection. He took decisive action, unwilling to leave such an important goal in his life to chance. I know it might be naïve to believe that everyone who works hard on it will become happily married, but your chances are certainly much better.

Remember that it is never too late to find a life partner, although the "conventional wisdom" might dictate otherwise. Who has ever gotten anywhere in life following the "conventional wisdom"? I recently prepared a prenuptial agreement for a female client who is seventy-eight years old. She was marrying for the fourth time. My mother is in her seventies and dating someone seriously.

Stoking the Fires of Passion

True love never grows old.

—Anonymous

Why buy the cow when you can get the milk for free?

—Anonymous

Don't Fret Our Love

Don't fret our love.
It's blessed from above.
We have our ways.

We'll have our days.
But the important thing
Is listening,
And feeling,
And talking,
And cutting each other some slack.
From arguments we'll bounce back,
Because the way we feel is very real.
My heart is yours.
Of that I am sure.
So don't fret our love.
It's blessed from above.

—Tim Burns

Keeping the passion alive is the greatest challenge of any relationship, particularly after the newness has worn off. In the groundbreaking book *The Road Less Traveled,* M. Scott Peck distinguishes between true love and infatuation, the latter being nature's way of perpetuating the species. It is no coincidence that this period of initial infatuation lasts approximately two years, which is about the time required to fall in love, get married, and then become pregnant. Afterwards, the couple must work to advance their infatuation up the slippery slope of their relationship to true love.

After that initial glow fades, the real work is required in the relationship. All the faults that were conveniently glossed over suddenly spring to the surface. As time passes, it can be tempting to take your spouse or significant other for granted and to put the relationship on cruise control. However, relationships require sustained work to maintain them. It can be easy, in today's obsession with instant gratification, to simply move on when the going gets tough. Couples find themselves falling out of love but then don't take action to address the issue. They may decide to remain together due to convenience or for the sake of their children. There may be legitimate reasons to split up, such as adultery, abuse, or alcoholism (or other substance abuse), which is also known as the three As. Less serious problems such as relationship drift or communication problems can be resolved with some work. A counselor friend of mine told me that even when couples are visibly angry with each other, there's still a chance for the relationship. But when they are completely apathetic towards each other, the relationship is in serious trouble.

An excellent book on sustaining passion in your relationship is entitled *50 Ways to Create Great Relationships: How to Stop Taking and Start Giving*. The author provides numerous techniques to keep the fires of passion alive. The bottom line is giving, giving, and then giving some more. Take the initiative to create a great relationship instead of simply reacting to your partner. Make it a habit to do something nice for your partner and set the stage for a harmonious relationship that creates passion. It also helps to avoid unnecessary conflict as well as the need to hold your ground on some trivial matter "for the principle of it." So what if your husband has a habit of leaving the cap off of the toothpaste or your wife never seems to have the proper directions? Although these are stereotypes, many pet peeves are the basis for unnecessary conflict. And was it all really worth it, the petty things that can escalate and cause marital discord?

Couples can also allow the passion to flicker out by failing to communicate, failing to express appreciation, and being emotionally distant from each other. Remember that the initial glow will always fade out, and that's when the real work starts. Instead, some people go from relationship to relationship, almost addicted to this initial glow. People become restless in their marriage. We all know people who have had multiple partners or even multiple marriages in their constant quest for passion. Perhaps they are seeking the perfect person, the one with whom the glow will not dim. But often the key is not to keep changing partners but to roll up your sleeves and work on the relationship.

Of course, there needs to be an adequate basis for the relationship. During the period of initial infatuation, many serious incompatibilities are concealed. Even two people who love each other need an adequate basis for companionship. Think of companionship as two circles. Each life is a separate circle, and the more the circles intersect, the more compatible the couple will be and the more common interests they will share. All the passion in the world is not going to assist a couple whose respective circles of life never intersect. In my earlier years, I would bury myself in projects for maybe months at a time while expecting the relationship to hum along without me. However, it just doesn't work that way, and it is very difficult to maintain the fire in the relationship if you're not spending significant quality time together. Think of it as forming a bond to resist that gravity pull of busy, over-stimulated lives. There are many distractions out there that could easily wreck a relationship. It is simply too easy to grow apart and begin looking again for something or someone else to light the fire. That is why extramarital affairs are common in this country. One spouse feels neglected and is looking for some attention.

Much of the work of spouses is to continually recreate this initial glow. That is why a date night is still important even for married couples. I served as a waiter for a number of years in a fine restaurant and could always tell the married couples from those who were dating. The gentlemen seemed much more attentive to their dates than husbands were to their wives. Occasionally, I would see a married couple who was physically affectionate and where the romance was obviously alive. But, unfortunately, this seems to be the exception rather than the rule.

Keeping the passion alive is not so much about buying expensive gifts but acting in spontaneous and unexpected ways. Society has, of course, mandated that we honor Valentine's Day. But taking the time to do little, unexpected things for your spouse or significant other on a regular basis can help retain the passion. One of the more interesting stories from *50 Ways to Create Great Relationships* was a gentleman dressing up in a tuxedo to deliver a flower to an old girlfriend on her birthday. When questioned by his roommate about such a curious act performed early on a Saturday morning, he replied that he simply wanted to do something special for her on her special day. They became married. Another person, who had been through a bitter divorce, put a note on his to-do list every day to do something nice for his current wife. He found that he neglected his previous relationship, and he did not want this one to follow the same unsuccessful path. Such little things can add up to a lot of passion.

Couples who are stuck in a loveless marriage are often faced with the difficult decision of whether or not to try to salvage the relationship. In many cases, the couple simply cannot live together for one reason or another. Constant turbulence can be a sign that the relationship is in trouble.

Many remain in loveless marriages because of the comfort level. They may need to try to reignite the passion or cut their losses with their relationship. Many people, including myself, are simply afraid of being alone. Many would settle for a less than ideal relationship rather than risk being alone. When I look back at my previous long-term relationship, I see that it was way too long. The passion had cooled, we had grown far apart, and we were staying together more out of codependency than true passion and love. Couples can find all kinds of excuses to stay together: financial, children, the inconvenience of divorce. As someone whose parents stayed together when perhaps they shouldn't have, I can say that it is much healthier to raise children in an atmosphere of mutual respect than in a turbulent environment where people are simply sharing the same roof. Deciding whether or not the relationship is irreparable can be very difficult, and sometimes it should be done with the assistance of professional counseling. There's often a fine line between beating a dead horse and reviving a relationship that is worth salvaging.

Your Purpose Is to Have a Great Relationship

But love is blind, and lovers cannot see
The pretty follies that themselves commit.
                                                        —Shakespeare

Everyone deserves a great relationship. Just like an unsatisfactory career, life is simply too short to be stuck in an unsatisfactory relationship. Often the question is whether or not a current relationship needs work and rejuvenation. As we will discuss in the next section, it is possible to tune up an existing relationship. However, the purpose and the commitment must be present.

Studies have shown that people are happiest when they are in committed relationships. They tend to live longer and have happier lives. However, you do have to be willing to lose yourself to some degree in a relationship and be willing to compromise. That is why it can be more difficult to enter into relationships later in life. People have become more "set in their ways" and are less willing to compromise. I see this inability to compromise in many of my friends who are divorced or still single. Rather than seeking the ideal spouse, find someone with whom you have complementary features and with whom you are compatible. As I wrote earlier, don't frustrate yourself searching for the Holy Grail. The truth is, although your mate might be out there, the perfect person is not. Don't forget that you are not perfect either.

Many people might consider themselves better off alone. In fact, being able to be alone can be an important prerequisite to a good relationship. This solitude can help you understand that your happiness is not necessarily dependent upon the actions of someone else. The time alone can help you decide what you want in a relationship and, more importantly, what you are ready to give. Some commentators have suggested today's generation doesn't really care enough to make the necessary sacrifices and behavior modifications to sustain a relationship. Good relationships aren't the priority they once were.

Unfortunately, not everyone who wants one is going to have a great relationship. I know that there are plenty of lonely people out there who have had their hearts broken and who have given up ever trying to find a suitable mate. I really hope you do and I hope that you don't give up. I wrote earlier about my mother, who suffered through a loveless marriage to later find true love in her fifties and then later again in her seventies. I knew of another woman with two teenage children whose husband died tragically from cancer. She would visit the cemetery every Sunday and noticed a gentleman there who was also visiting a deceased spouse. One day, the man began to cry, and she walked over and asked if she could help. He said that her voice reminded him of an angel. They started dating and eventually married. So if you don't have that primary relationship that you are looking for, please don't give up hope. There's always hope, provided you allow it to come into your life.

Many people confuse having a great relationship with fulfilling their personal needs. Great relationships involve compromise and giving. If you simply want companionship and a clean house, maybe you should buy a dog and hire a housekeeper.

According to noted author M. Scott Peck, love is the giving

of yourself for the spiritual development of another. Such an unselfish attitude forms the basis for a good relationship. Many who have not had their emotional needs fixed are simply looking for someone to fix them. They keep hopping from relationship to relationship, hoping to find the one that does the trick. The truth is that no one can fix you. You are the only one who can fix yourself. Although your spouse should be supportive of you, the purpose of a romantic relationship is not to fix you. That is *your* job. But after you've fixed yourself the best that you can, you'll be in a position to give yourself for the spiritual development of another.

Empowering Your Relationship

> We don't love qualities, we love a person; sometimes by reason of their defects as well as their qualities.
> —Jacques Maritain, *Reflections on America*

As stated earlier, giving of yourself is the best way to empower a relationship. But not everyone follows this advice. Sometimes they are narcissistic and simply don't take the time to give. But if you are going to empower your relationship, you need to make your relationship a priority in your life. Don't expect a good relationship if it is a distant second to your work or personal needs. When two people join together with the common goal of supporting the spiritual development of the other, they create an environment in which a relationship can thrive. Don't think of such giving as compromising but instead as synchronizing to create a stronger union and a better life for both of you.

It is not just the quantity of time but also the quality of time spent that empowers the relationship. Forgiveness and empathy can also serve to empower relationships. People tend to cling to their positions. Remember that there are two sides to every story, and even if it is 60/40 in your favor, what is the point? Resolve to forgive and forget, and focus on the relationship. Although it often takes courage to admit that you're wrong, it's well worth it.

Qualities that can assist in empowering your relationship include empathy, understanding, communication, and commitment. Empathy is the ability to consider another's point of view. The old saying is that you have to walk in another's moccasins before passing judgment. There is much wisdom in this statement. Too often we become rigid about our own point of view and don't take the time to consider where someone else is "coming from." Innocent remarks are frequently misinterpreted and become the basis for disputes. If someone begins a sentence with the phrase "when you do or say this, I feel . . . " they are being nonjudgmental and speaking from their heart about how your actions affect them. Instead of becoming instantly defensive, try to understand where they are coming from. How can you fault someone for feeling a certain way? If your spouse is upset about something, don't take it as a personal attack but simply an expression of their feelings. Rather than becoming offended, try to empathize with their feelings. If you do, there is a much better chance of working out the dispute.

Empathy is very closely related to understanding. It can be difficult to try to understand someone and take the time to legitimize their feelings. Sometimes people are simply "venting" because they just want to be heard and understood. I find that men, who often try to be problem solvers, become unnerved when women express frustration, because men don't know how to react. "What do you want me to do about it?" they ask. The answer may be, "Nothing but listen, and legitimize my feelings."

Poor communication skills are probably the leading cause of failure in relationships. Couples who don't communicate their feelings and desires often grow apart. Effective communication skills include listening as well as expressing your feelings. In today's hectic world, many couples spend little time on quality communication. Listening involves really listening—eliminating every distraction around you, including your own thoughts of what you might say or do next, to really hear and also feel what the other person is saying. Effective listening also involves learning to be present in the relationship. Are you present for your spouse or significant other? Poor listening skills erect barriers to effective communication. If someone is always ignored, it simply becomes too frustrating to communicate anymore. Although I wrote earlier about the benefits of therapy, some are paying therapists just because they need someone to listen and acknowledge their feelings. The greatest gifts you can give another are your time and undivided attention, to let them know beyond a shadow of a doubt that their feelings, thoughts, and issues are important to you. There is no better way to empower your relationship than to listen.

Another important way to empower your relationship is through a spiritual practice. With a national divorce rate over 50 percent, couples who attend religious services together reduce their divorce rates to an astonishing 5 percent. In addition, the divorce rate of couples who pray together is less than 3 percent. Today, relationships can be so challenging that they require the constant help, supervision, and involvement of God. In his book entitled *Three to Get Married,* Archbishop Fulton Sheen points out that God often is a necessary third party in a successful marriage. It's interesting that, in my previous long-term relationship that fizzled out, we did not attend religious services together. However, attending religious services together is an important part of my current relationship.

Planning to Boost Your Relationship

It's an extra dividend when you like the girl that you're in love with.

—Clark Gable

Assessment. The first step in improving your relationship is assessing it. Why do people flounder along without their needs being met when an average relationship can be turned into a great relationship? According to Gestalt psychology, there are many subtle influences on our choice of a mate, such as family-of-origin issues. A principle in Gestalt is that most people tend to identify with one parent and then marry the other parent. A very wise counselor once illustrated for me the influence of our childhood on relationships, which actually consists of three forces.

- Parent: both the positive and negative traits we acquired from our parents.
- Adult: the rational adult self that makes decisions.
- Child: could involve our unmet needs as a child and could result in our overreacting to certain situations or reacting as a child would.

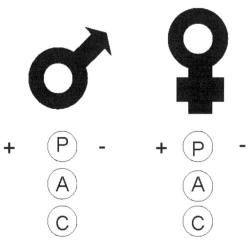

The counselor gave me the example of a couple where the wife would tend to lash out when angry or upset about something her husband did or usually forgot to do. She'd had a strict upbringing in which she suffered verbal abuse for not finishing her chores. However, her anger would make her husband withdraw and do less, since his background made him very averse to conflict. This would lead to more anger from his wife, who felt ignored, and he would withdraw more, feeling attacked. The escalation of their anger over often trivial matters clearly involved little of their adult selves but mostly negative influences from their parents and childish reactions.

By understanding the dynamics, they then became able to nip most conflicts in the bud. She was more diplomatic about undone chores and realized she could catch more flies with honey than vinegar. He responded better to gentle coaxing.

This model provides hope that anyone who is in love and committed can work through practically anything. Because of negative influences from our youth, couples can blow small things out of proportion. Once they can assess and contain the cause of much of their conflict, a potentially combustible, stressful situation can reach a rational conclusion. With this approach, it is possible to remove much of the conflict from our lives.

If a relationship is in trouble, professional counseling can be a good option. Sometimes, it takes a trained professional to cut through the emotional clutter that may be interfering with your relationship. However, you can make a relationship work if you are honest in assessing the problems and willing to commit to the relationship.

Planning. A plan to boost your relationship involves working through the differences, forgetting past behavior, and even recommitting to your partner. But don't wait for your partner to take the initiative. Resolve to take the initiative and begin giving yourself to the relationship. Often you will find that your commitment and effort are returned.

Reexamining your primary relationship—your relationship with your spouse or significant other—may be your most difficult midlife assessment. I must confess that I could probably tell you more what not to do than what to do in this area. In many cases, it is helpful to go through the same steps as for an emotional tune-up, including forgiveness. We have all made mistakes in a primary relationship. Many of us had very unrealistic expectations about what it was supposed to be. My role model for a primary relationship was so bad I didn't want one. I had to come to grips with that and realize that not all primary relationships were like my parents'.

The emotional baggage discussed earlier affects your primary relationship. Often, if you take care of your emotional baggage, your attitude about relationships will improve. One of the main symptoms of a midlife crisis is a lack of interest in a primary relationship and a desire to seek outside excitement or fulfillment, usually through an illicit affair. This can be a very destructive and compulsive behavior.

The bottom line is that relationships, like everything else, take a lot of work. It never ceases to amaze me how people spend time on hobbies or nothing at all, yet they will not think of going to any type of course to improve their relationship. Many religious organizations sponsor "encounter weekends" and other programs to strengthen primary relationships. Few people attend such workshops because it sounds like too much trouble. But how much trouble is a bad relationship? Isn't it worth investing some time in the person with whom you are sharing your life? Many people who spend hours of their time on continuing education or exercising at the gym are unwilling to commit time to their primary relationship.

Perspective in Long-Term Relationships

Retaining a proper perspective in your long-term relationship is very much a key to ensuring its ultimate success. A couple's happiness needs to be judged not necessarily on their honeymoon but on their fiftieth anniversary.

Spiritual guidance can be an important element in preserving a long-term relationship. But a good way to preserve your relationship is not necessarily the golden rule: do unto others as you would have them do unto you. Instead, do unto others as they wish to be done to. That involves empathy and the selflessness and insight to put yourself in another person's shoes.

As a good friend of mine who is looking to get remarried stated, she wants somebody to last for the long haul. We have to decide what traits we can live with and what others would be a significant impediment to a long-term relationship. But don't necessarily count on people changing. Generally, people resent being asked to change, and suddenly being told that their behavior is unacceptable rarely leaves them feeling positive. Instead, you have to make a realistic assessment about whether or not you can live with that person. One down side to trying to change somebody is that once you change them they're really not the same person you were interested in in the first place. Don't think that you can get into a relationship, change the person, and then everything will be fine. Understand that whether or not the relationship will lose depends on the couple's ability to adapt, grow, and change together while retaining perspective in the relationship.

Perseverance in Your Relationship

Making relationships last obviously requires a lot of effort. It wasn't that long ago that divorce was a grave step and most people stayed in relationships as opposed to going through the trouble of getting a divorce. Now most states allow no-fault divorces and have made the dissolving of marital unions quite easy. The pendulum might have swung too far and made it too easy for people to dissolve potentially viable relationships rather than work on them. Louisiana, among other states, has started what is known as a covenant marriage, which legally binds the couple to counseling before they decide to dissolve the marriage. It imposes a legal requirement for perseverance. I wish everyone the best of luck with their relationships. If you're in a relationship, I hope you can work to make it a great one. If you're not, I sincerely hope and pray that you find the person you're looking for, that you obtain the love you deserve, and that your perseverance pays off.

I had basically given up on ever getting married until I met Karen. As I mentioned earlier, I had been soured by a long-term relationship that ended on an unproductive note. I think I spent much of my time "hanging around" in comfortable relationships that best fit my lifestyle. I had no interest in moving farther up the relationship ladder, because it distracted me from other pursuits. Looking back, I see I just wasn't willing to really give of myself.

All of that changed almost instantly when I met Karen. There was a deep attraction and then I quickly fell in love. As our infatuation moved to love, I was forced to finally confront all of the issues about relationships that I preached about earlier in the chapter. It wasn't easy. It required that I change my entire paradigm of relationships and confront not only relationship issues but unresolved family-of-origin issues. The wise counselor told me that we tend to pair up with those who make us address unresolved childhood issues.

But I persevered, and as someone who stayed single while his sister and his cousins married, and was still single while the children of his cousins married, I finally took my own advice and got married as well. If I can tune up my approach to my primary relationship, then you can, too.

CHAPTER 15

Physical Tune-Up

Falstaff sweats to death
And lards the lean earth as he walks along.

—Shakespeare

I have more flesh than another man, and therefore more frailty.

—Shakespeare

Despite living in the most affluent society in the world, with medical breakthroughs occurring practically on a daily basis, Americans are in the midst of a serious health crisis. Currently, 60 percent of adults, approximately 97 million people, are considered overweight or obese. Over 300,000 people die each year from obesity-related illnesses alone. In addition, there has been a one-third increase in diabetes, which can be attributed to a lack of exercise and being overweight. Over 10 percent of people living United States suffer from severe fatigue, which is rooted in physiological causes that are completely avoidable.

Unfortunately, our response has been either to do nothing or go on yo-yo diets (constantly losing then finding those pesky pounds). However, the real answer is to make healthy, permanent lifestyle changes that include proper diet and exercise. This will increase both the quality and quantity of our years.

Physical Tune-Up Can Create Passion

There is no quicker way to improve your outlook, stamina, and well-being than a physical tune-up, which includes proper nutrition, exercise, and rest.

Simply put, proper nutrition includes those items located at the perimeter of your grocery store ("The Good") and avoids or limits many of the foods in the middle ("The Bad"). In other words, consume more fresh fruits, vegetables, lean meats, poultry, fish, grains, and, and lean dairy products and less processed foods, beef, sweets, and frozen pizza. Also avoid excess caffeine and alcohol and refrain from tobacco use.

Regular exercise should include both aerobic and strength-conditioning activities. A forty-five-minute exercise routine three to five times a week can produce significant health benefits. Since the benefits of exercise tend to taper off once you get started, you can obtain good results from just a moderate exercise regimen.

The final ingredient of a physical tune-up is rest. We all need a certain amount of it in order to function at our best. Determine the amount of rest that you need, which is usually eight to nine hours a night, and then resolve to get it.

A proper diet, exercise routine, and sufficient rest are all key ingredients for physical passion in your life. I found that I was best able to deal with life, particularly those stressful periods, when I followed a proper health regimen. Physical activity releases endorphins, which results in a natural feeling of wellness. The runner's high, which you may have heard about, does exist and can provide a tremendous energy boost. I've experienced it many times, not only from running but also from other cardiovascular exercise. A physical tune-up helps to stir the passion in our soul as well as enhances our outlook and performance. Nothing makes you feel better on the inside than creating a new you on the outside. Proper diet and exercise can dramatically reshape your appearance, increase your energy, and improve your attitude. Take the time to increase your effectiveness, happiness, and life span with a physical tune-up.

Your Purpose Is Adopting a Healthy Lifestyle

Nations have passed away and left no traces,
And history gives the naked causes of it—
One single, simple reason in all cases;
They fell because their people were not fit.

—Rudyard Kipling, *Land and Sea Tales*
for Scouts and Guides

People tend to take their health for granted until they lose it. Unfortunately, by that time, it may be too late. Although we all have genetic predispositions to certain illnesses, we can significantly enhance our health with proper diet and exercise. According to the American Cancer Society, the risk of even the most dreaded disease in our society can be significantly lessened with—you guessed it—proper diet and exercise. So why do so many of us ignore such evidence that favors a healthy lifestyle? As with many life changes, people have a difficult time "just getting started." Although it can be easy to be overwhelmed by the information and choices available, adopting a healthy lifestyle involves just a few changes to your daily routine that can pay tremendous returns.

All experts agree that becoming physically fit can add many quality years to your life. Start by asking yourself: How do I feel? How do I look? Have I had a full physical and are there some potential health issues that can be addressed now?

Your purpose is not to be a champion athlete or, depending on your gender, a muscle man or spandex model. Instead, your purpose is the permanent adoption of healthy lifestyle choices, primarily through proper diet and exercise. Many are intimidated by gyms and even the thought of changing their physical routine. Some boomers might feel reluctant to expose themselves physically to the younger folks. However, there are many fitness solutions for time-pressured people. I recently advised a legal client on her investment in a Curves franchise. My review of the offering documents led me to realize what a powerful and necessary service they provide in the marketplace. Curves features a circuit-training program for women and offers a regimented routine that is designed to make physical fitness more convenient and affordable. I understand that Cuts is opening as a franchise for men. These are just some of the options for regular exercise. Gyms, YMCA, and facilities associated with health plans or other health clubs are springing up across the country. The YMCA (as well as YWCA) does have a policy of only charging people what they can afford. So if your budget is tight, it is a viable option. You can also purchase equipment for your home. Remember that you can realize tremendous benefits with a moderate exercise routine. Along with a proper diet, this can assist in your quest for permanent, healthy lifestyle changes.

Empower Yourself with a
Proper Diet and Exercise

Fatigue makes cowards of us all.

—Vince Lombardi

Proper diet. The foundation of a proper diet includes low-glycemic carbohydrates, lean proteins, acceptable fat, as well as fiber. The chart below lists the acceptable and the less acceptable food groups. Contrary to popular belief, proper nutrition is not that difficult. Here is a recap of some of the more important elements.

- Avoid heavy intakes of caffeine and refined sugars.
- Avoid processed foods.
- Eat more fresh fruits and vegetables.
- Eat fish and lean meat.

Although fad diets try to make this process complicated, it doesn't have to be. Simply replace the fatty foods and refined sugars with complex carbohydrates and proteins. Eat more fruits and vegetables and try to avoid anything that comes in a cellophane package. For those of us on the go, meal replacements such as energy bars and nutrient drinks can be good sources of healthy nutrition. In the best-selling book *Body for Life,* fitness guru Bill Phillips recommends eating one portion of complex carbohydrates and one portion of proteins six times per day. Although I found eating six times a day a bit difficult, I do usually try to graze throughout the day. It is important to avoid big meals, particularly at the latter part of the day, as those calories tend to stick to you. Find those foods out there that help you to stick to your routine, such as cottage cheese and/or tuna fish with a slice of wheat bread. The key is simplicity. Develop the habit of eating the right things. Once you get in the habit, it becomes second nature.

Another diet book, which originated in my hometown, is *SugarBusters!* which advocated the avoidance of refined sugar as well as unrefined sugar in any form. Their regimen is very strict, extending beyond simple sweets to include such items as bananas and carrots.

Many have had success with the Atkins Diet, which totally avoids any carbohydrates and allows for saturated fats, such as bacon, pork rinds, and sausage. But this diet is at odds with some others that urge a more modified approach to carbohydrates. I know some who started on the Atkins Diet and achieved some results and then gradually began adding carbohydrates back into their diet.

A summary of suggested diets appears below. Note that it recommends more of the important food groups such as complex carbohydrates, protein, non-saturated fat, and fiber ("The Good") and less of the bad carbohydrates, saturated fat, and refined sugars ("The Bad"). And, of course, you want to moderate your alcohol and caffeine use and refrain from tobacco use ("The Ugly"). Don't try to be perfect in your diet, but make healthy choices as much as possible.

Exercise. You can also empower yourself with exercise. As with dieting, I have been most successful with exercise when I have gotten into a routine. Find an exercise activity that appeals to you, whether it be cycling, running, or aerobics classes, and work it into your routine. Nothing is more satisfying than finishing a workout and being empowered by that energy.

Dieting 101

Important Food Groups	The Good	The Bad	The Ugly
Complex Carbohydrates	Fresh vegetables, particularly anything green	(Saturated fats, refined sugars and bad carbohydrates)	Tobacco (in any form)
	Fresh fruit, particularly apples, blueberries, blackberries, cherries, oranges and peaches	-beef -white bread -muffins	Alcohol (more than a moderate amount)
Protein	Fresh fish, tuna, mackerel, salmon	-pancakes -refined sugar -table sugar	
	Lean meats, fat free cottage cheese, turkey, tuna	-jam -butter	
	Low fat milk, soy milk and products	-candy -cheese	
Non-Saturated Fat	Vegetable oil, nuts, avocados		
Fiber	Nuts, beans, peas, lentils, brown rice, raw fruits		

Plan Your Physical Tune-Up

As discussed earlier, a physical tune-up is less about fad diets and sporadic activity and more about committing to a lifestyle change. Most New Year's resolutions fall by the wayside because their focus is short term (lose ten pounds), while a lifestyle change is long term. Instead of focusing on losing the weight, or denying yourself, the key is to focus upon changing your lifestyle. As opposed to going on a crash diet and exercise program for a few weeks, take gradual steps that you can incorporate permanently into your lifestyle.

In the previous section, we discussed the optimal diet choices. But don't view your diet from the standpoint of denial, that you are giving up so many things that you love. Instead, consider your diet from a positive standpoint, that you are adding healthier, leaner foods to your diet such as fish and vegetables. Such foods are anti-carcinogens as well as healthier.

We live in a busy society. Many of us don't have the time to prepare meals that perfectly match the above chart. However, once you develop a routine, you can make the time. Instead of driving to a fast-food restaurant window, take some fruits and vegetables with you in the morning. I carry apples and pears with me as well as the lean carbohydrate bars. Healthy diets are often built upon small choices, such as avoiding heavy salad dressings, substituting skim milk for whole milk, ordering grilled items instead of fried, ordering fish and poultry instead of steak, and so on. Although fresh vegetables have more nutrients, it is not always possible to eat them. If you sometimes have to eat frozen or canned vegetables, then do so. They are still better for you than the wrong types of foods. You can't always eat perfectly, so do the best that you can with what you have. The idea is to keep veering towards the proper lifestyle choice. If you do, the pounds will come off, your energy will grow, you will feel better, and, more importantly, you will extend your life.

When planning your lifestyle change, don't try to overdo it. Your plan does not need to include joining a health club, hiring a personal trainer, hiring a dietitian, and obsessively following a brand-new diet all at the same time. While all of these steps are of course positive, I find that if you set modest goals and pursue them, you are much better off. A recent study of 25,000 dieting people found that most lost weight not through particular groups but through dieting on their own.

We have also discussed the benefits of exercise. It can help you in so many different areas. Exercise not only makes you feel better physically and mentally but also helps to curb your appetite. The key is to be realistic, find a physical activity that you are inclined to do, work it into your routine, and stay consistent. If you have never exercised before, it might help to use a personal trainer. And if you can afford it, schedule at least five or ten sessions as opposed to just one. One meeting with a fitness trainer to set up your routine will not give you enough momentum. You generally need five to ten sessions to really get your routine down. And the more regularly you follow your routine, the more likely you are to stick to it. I know this from my personal experience. Over the years, I have scheduled single sessions on a sporadic basis. Finally, a trainer I befriended urged me to schedule ten sessions. I gulped a bit but followed his advice, which did help me get into a routine and produced excellent results.

It is not always necessary to hire a fitness trainer. You might instead want to ask some of the fitness consultants at the clubs for their help. The quality of their assistance can vary vastly, depending upon their experience and their interest in helping you.

An exercise plan should involve both a weight-training regimen and cardiovascular exercise. Some clubs offer a circuit-training routine, which combines aerobic and strength training. Such workouts are broken into thirty-minute segments and are designed for busy people. But if you stick to a routine, the benefits will begin to roll in. Avoid socializing too much; maximize your time at your gym. Give each session your best without overexerting yourself, and even try to enjoy it a little. Don't attack every piece of equipment and wind up getting too sore to exercise. Your goal is not immediate results but a gradual transformation.

An important element of exercise is strength training. Studies have shown that stronger muscles tend to last longer and produce strong bones. In addition, strength training can be very restorative. I had a nagging condition with a hamstring for a number of years that actually prevented me from running, the cardiovascular activity of my choice. It wasn't until I worked with a personal trainer and began doing leg lifts that I was able to break down the scar tissue in the muscle and finally experience pain-free running. Resistance training also slows down the aging process. However, be sure to take the time to stretch before every workout.

Although most trainers recommend free weights, the Nautilus-type equipment can be a good start for the novice. The key is proper technique. Avoid using exercise equipment until you have proper instruction. Otherwise, you can waste a lot of time and risk injury with improper usage. Posture, breathing, and proper technique combine to provide the most benefits. Do not sacrifice technique for weight. Men in particular try to measure their progress by how much they can lift on various equipment. However, it is not necessarily the weight that you lift but the maximum you can do with proper technique that matters. Are you benefiting from resistance in both parts of the exercise? Are you focusing on pushing the weight out but not also on the resistance coming back? If so, you could be missing as much as half of the benefits of the exercise.

If you do not have the resources to join a health club, check out the YMCA, as I mentioned earlier. Branches are found in just about every city and they are very flexible with their fees. If you have never exercised before, I strongly recommend joining some type of club. That way you can get properly instructed in a program. It is much better to find someone knowledgeable to work with you than chance it on your own.

Maintaining Perspective in the Physical Tune-Up

One of the most intimidating prospects in visiting a gym is viewing all the hard, lean bodies sweating away. I know that it was very easy for me to become intimidated. However, remember that the only person against whom you are measuring your progress is you. Stick to your exercise routine and you will eventually begin to feel and notice the benefits. The same perspective applies to diet. Don't compare yourself to others. Measure your progress in steady, incremental goals. Just like your finances, you are investing in your body, the only one that you get. Don't become discouraged; understand that it takes weeks and even months to fully realize the benefits of a healthy lifestyle.

The more that you can work proper diet and exercises into

your existing routine, the more likely they will become a permanent part of your life. Our available time for exercise is generally dictated by the other demands on us. I find that exercising in the morning gives me more energy for the rest of the day. By the time I "wake up," my workout is almost over. Others might find that the evening is a more flexible time for their workout. Women might need more time to prepare themselves in the morning. Often, when I was involved in a major project, such as writing a book or running a campaign, my workouts would stop. This generally would make me antsy and I would have to get to the gym to "get my head on straight." I found that there was nothing better for starting the day with a clear focus than a morning workout. It put me in the proper frame of mind for the rest of the day. I feel better now and have more energy than I did fifteen years ago. Much of this is due to the fact that I've changed my lifestyle.

The following advice from the American Health Foundation provides a good way to maintain perspective in your physical tune-up:

Ten Golden Rules for Good Health

1. Have a checkup every year.
2. Be a nonsmoker.
3. Drink in moderation.
4. Count each calorie.
5. Watch your cholesterol.
6. Learn nutritional values.
7. Find time for leisure and vacations.
8. Adjust to life's daily pressures.
9. Develop an exercise program.
10. Understand your physical assets and limitations.

Perseverance with Physical Health

Patience and perseverance have a magical effect before which difficulties disappear and obstacles vanish.

—John Quincy Adams

Few things require more perseverance than sticking to an exercise and diet regimen. As someone who's been going to health clubs for a number of years, I can report that they

always fill up in the first month of the year with people looking to remake their bodies. During that time, I would go in
the early morning to avoid the evening rush. But usually by
the end of January, attendance is back to normal. Most New
Year's resolutions have petered out by that time. Although
the regulars are still there, many of the newcomers have
dropped out, their only contact with the gym being the monthly debit from their checking account. The same applies to
diets. I have friends who are constantly starting diets. That is
because they never finished the last diet that they started. If
they persevered, they would not always be starting diets but
instead would be maintaining their ideal body weight.
Persevere with your lifestyle change of healthier eating and
moderate exercise. It may take a while before you notice the
benefits, but they will come, and they will extend both the
quality and quantity of your years.

CHAPTER 16

Mental Tune-Up

A little learning is a dangerous thing;
Drink deep, or taste not the Pierian spring;
There shall draughts intoxicate the brain,
And drinking largely sobers us again.
> —Alexander Pope, "An Essay on Criticism"

Develop a Passion for Learning

As our society plunges deeper into the Information Age, the value of knowledge cannot be overstated. We all know how rapidly technology and processes are changing, making it necessary to keep feeding our minds with new ideas and information. Numerous sources of information, from books to cassettes, CDs, the Internet, and other media outlets, can both assist and overwhelm us at the same time. Still, we live in an exciting time. So don't be intimidated by the information explosion. Instead, develop a passion for learning. This doesn't mean that you have to master every new gizmo as it hits the market, but be open to learning the most important changes and information.

Lifelong Learning Is Your Purpose

Learning is a treasure which accompanies its owner everywhere.

> —Chinese proverb

Similar to the physical tune-up, the mental tune-up involves a lifelong commitment. In order to keep my knowledge base current, I read several periodicals as well as between fifty and seventy-five books annually. Now don't gasp, since this is not as impossible as it sounds. I skim through most of the periodicals, first checking the table of contents to determine which articles are of particular interest. I focus on those articles and generally skim the rest. If an article is important enough, I'll tear it out and then scan it into my computer. With regards to books, my secret weapon is audiocassettes and CDs. Most of the books I "read" I actually listen to in my car. I find audio learning to be quite convenient, as I can obtain the benefits while I am doing something else, like driving. I subscribe to one service that sends me, on a monthly basis, condensed versions of two leading business books on audio tape. That is about one-third of my book goal right there. The other tapes I either order or rent from the library or rental outlets.

Another secret to lifelong learning is using your down time productively. You'd be surprised how this time accumulates and how much you can learn during these intervals. I know I was. Time spent waiting for appointments or at the airport can be used productively. And, of course, if you drive a lot, turn your car into a rolling university. Listen to inspirational and educational audio tapes.

Learning = Power

> Knowledge is power.
>
> —Anonymous

> Education is simply the soul of a society as it passes from one generation to another.
> —G. K. Chesterton, *The Observer,* "Sayings of the Week"

> You must learn day by day, year by year, to broaden your horizon. The more things you love, the more you are interested in, the more you enjoy, the more you are indignant about—the more you have left when something happens.
> —Ethel Barrymore

Don't ever underestimate the extent to which you can empower yourself with learning. Fortunes have been made and empires launched on the strength of a single new idea. Often such ideas were inspired by new information. That is why it is so important to remain mentally alert and open to new information, which doesn't necessarily have to be academic or business information. My grandmother stayed mentally alert by playing cards. Keep current in your areas of interest and hobbies as well as your career. Read or absorb anything that keeps your mind active. Continually challenge yourself and keep growing mentally.

Expertise or knowledge is obviously the main currency in the information economy. First and foremost, you need to be an authority in your career in order to succeed. Note that I did not say well read or extremely knowledgeable. I said an authority. As we discussed earlier, in the career chapter, it is possible to become an authority by committing yourself to your career for just one hour a day.

The knowledge demands of your career can be particularly fierce, and it is often difficult to handle the flow of information that is relevant to your business. Trade journals, magazines, newspapers, newsletters, and other sources of information seem to cascade over your desk on a regular basis. And that's not even counting the online world, with its infinite world of electronic information.

In addition to career and personal items, there is much information available in the area of peak performance or motivation that can help with your life. One of the pioneers of the self-help movement was Dale Carnegie, whose self-development programs enhanced personal interaction skills. His classic book, *How to Win Friends and Influence People,* was a precursor to many of today's relationship skills and personal effectiveness programs. Numerous other self-help gurus have come along since Carnegie. Dr. Wayne Dyer instructs us on how to be a "no limit" person. Tony Robbins advocates the use of neurolinguistic programming or NLP in order to communicate more effectively with others. Dr. Steven Covey instructs us about the seven habits of highly effective people. Deepak Chopra equips us with strategies to combat aging and tap into the collective wisdom of the universe.

Much of the material espoused by these self-help gurus as well as other motivational speakers is based on timeless wisdom, management development strategies, and common sense. The authors put their own spin on the material, with some interpretations being more unique and successful than others. Some of the self-help strategies I studied were too simplistic as well as overhyped. Problems don't just disappear because you have a good attitude or have gained some knowledge about them. Although knowledge can be power, you need to devise an effective mental tune-up plan that focuses on the information that is most important to your personal development.

Developing Your Lifelong Learning Plan

The development of a lifelong learning plan involves making an assessment of the knowledge necessary to benefit your career and life and then planning a strategy to keep current and learn those items of value.

Here are five important steps in developing your lifelong learning plan.

1. Focus on the areas you need to learn in: career, personal, self-development.
2. Dedicate one hour each day to learning. Sometimes the evening can be a good time for this, swapping out television and mindless Internet surfing for important personal enrichment.
3. Watch educational programming when it is available.
4. Attend at least one seminar/trade show annually in your most important field or endeavor.
5. Use audio materials and condensations to leverage downtime and maximize your time.

Maintaining Perspective in Your Learning

Education made us what we are.
—Claude-Adrien Helvetius, *Discours XXX*

Learning without thought is labor lost; thought without learning is perilous.
—Confucius, *The Analects*

Wisdom comes only through suffering.
—Aeschylus, *Agamemnon*

It is better to learn late than never.
—Anonymous

A fool at forty is a fool indeed.

—Anonymous

One way to maintain perspective in your learning is to be selective and avoid being overwhelmed. We have discussed earlier the literally infinite sources of information available. I know firsthand about being overwhelmed by information, as I must confess that I am a recovering "information addict." As with any problem of this sort, my "information addiction" started quite innocently and then quickly got out of hand. In response to solicitations, I ordered a few books here and a few magazines there. This, of course, resulted in even more solicitations. I ordered more material and the downward spiral continued. Before long, I was on every gold-plated, "this guy will buy anything" customer list. Solicitations poured in and even followed me around as I changed addresses. I found myself immersed in too much information. I needed to step back, refocus, and reprioritize.

Remember that you can't possibly read everything, so be selective with your information choices. Focus on the sources of information that are most important to your career and your life. And even be selective within those sources. No one ever said that you had to read a magazine cover to cover. Look at the table of contents and decide ahead of time which articles are most important. Read those carefully and then skim the rest. Usually your trade periodicals are more important than general business news. You might come across a very important article that you might want to save for future reference. Prioritize the information that you can get to and then ignore the rest.

Being selective about the material you read results in focusing on the things that truly matter. Not all information is created equal. Some information is much more important than others. Sometimes it is better to reread a particularly good piece of information than to read something new.

Maintaining perspective also involves setting up a good method of information retrieval. For years I saved printed information, which in many cases seemed to create more clutter than retrievable data. I then found scanners to be very useful in digitizing information. I was much more prone to use information that I had ready access to.

Persevere in Learning

Although it can be tedious, persevere in your quest for learning throughout your entire life. All great artists are practicing their crafts and even learning up until their very deaths. So persevere, and continue with learning. Don't be overwhelmed by the overflow of technology and information. Just resolve to stick to your learning plan.

CHAPTER 17

Spiritual Tune-Up

Know first, the heaven, the earth, the main,
The moon's pale orb, the starry train,
Are nourished by a soul,
A bright intelligence, whose flame
Glows in each member of the frame,
And stirs the mighty whole.

—Virgil

Developing a Passion for Regular Spiritual Practice

I have taught business courses at the college level for a number of years. One of my business law classes discussed the origin and evolution of the legal system in the United States. When I reread documents written by the Founding Fathers of this country who helped to write our Constitution, I was struck quite squarely by their religious nature. Our Founding Fathers were all very bright people who came together to create a government that has become the model for democracy in the world and made this nation a superpower. Their foresight and understanding of what didn't work in other governmental structures led them to create a system that we all (myself included) can complain about but that is still better than any other form of government in our world.

Our gifted founders were quick to acknowledge the relationship between our Creator and the government. Even though the Constitution included a separation between church and state in order to prevent religious persecution, our Founding Fathers made no secret of the fact that they were inspired by God. They formed a government based upon a doctrine of individual human rights bestowed upon every person by their Creator. In short, our country was created on a spiritual foundation, which led to the creation and

233

preservation of individual liberties. The doctrine "All men are created equal and endowed by their creator with certain inalienable rights" is a cornerstone of our society today. The founders acknowledged that the Creator endowed the government with power and that this is the only reason that government and other institutions exist.

As spirituality forms the foundation of our country, it should also form the foundation of your own life. In this sense I have saved the best for last, because the real path to serenity is through a spiritual tune-up. The common denominator among those who can handle adversity, who are genuinely happy, who live life to its fullest, and who lead moral lives is generally a spiritual foundation. In *The Road Less Traveled,* Dr. Peck writes about grace being available and abundant and humans being inherently spiritual creatures. However, people do not always respond to the spirituality that is there for the taking. They often ignore it.

I was raised as a Roman Catholic and attended parochial schools. Catholicism had a very strong influence on me. As a young adult, I kept going to church even though I did not feel like doing so. I did it mainly because my grandmother would always ask me if I did, and I could not lie to my grandmother. But even then, I viewed it as doing my time, a spiritual quid pro quo, a task I had to do in order to ask for things, as if God was keeping a giant ledger account upstairs. I would sit while the priest droned on, looking at my watch impatiently until I could go about doing "more important things."

I found that I only became deeply religious when I was very scared about something, trying to make a grade, looking for something, pursuing a certain goal, or facing a particular problem. It wasn't until I was in my thirties that I really began to appreciate religion in my life. It was when I realized that the important slogan "let go and let God" was deeply spiritual and how it could help me. Now I was attending mass not out of obligation but for enrichment. That is the point of a regular spiritual practice, to be spiritually enriched.

Regardless of your religion or whether you even have an institutional religion, it is important to maintain a spiritual basis in your life. When I was growing up, one of my favorite albums was by a band called Jethro Tull. It contained a song called "My God," which discussed the constraints that institutional religion sometimes places on the Creator.

Consequently, I am advocating a regular spiritual practice more than any type of religion. My spiritual practice happens to take place in the Roman Catholic Church, where I remain today.

Many use organized religion as a means of engaging in a regular spiritual practice. The structure and fellowship help to guide their spiritual renewal. Others approach their spiritual practice more individually. What is important is taking the time to contemplate or meditate and putting yourself in contact with your Higher Power, yourself, and the world. A regular spiritual practice can help rid your mind of clutter and negative thoughts. It can help sustain you, particularly during times of high stress. Not only can a regular spiritual practice produce inner peace, but it also can produce strength to draw from during times of adversity.

One of the most powerful experiences I ever had was a three-day silent retreat at the Manresa House of Retreats. It allows you to really get in touch with your inner self and your spiritual side. Much of what we do and worry about is all on the surface. We go running to and fro each day, dealing with the superficialities of life. The internal, fundamental items are often lost in the shuffle. It is that spiritual dimension that is so important to everyday life.

During my retreat at Manresa, I received a startling insight. Their motto is: "No one speaks to each other, but everyone speaks to God." It was no accident that I made a key emotional breakthrough during a spiritual exercise, because emotional health and spirituality are closely related. Many recovery programs, such as Alcoholic Anonymous, are spiritually based. Prayer can be a potent way to rid yourself of emotional baggage and provide the insight necessary to restore your passion.

The Manresa retreat consisted of lectures, prayer, and free time for meditation and even exercise. The message I received concerned my drinking. I had just finished jogging on the beautiful grounds and was stretching my legs on the fountain outside the retreat house when God spoke to me. His voice was unmistakable and filled my head with a quite pointed message. I could keep playing my cat-and-mouse game with alcohol, and it probably wouldn't kill me or send me to the gutter anytime soon. But I would never be as successful as I could be in life. That is because deep down I would know that

I was cheating. If I could cheat on myself on such a critical issue, with something that I knew was not good for me, that could easily get out of control, and that had ruined the lives of two grandfathers and my father, then I could cheat on other issues too. In other words, my willingness to accept mediocrity with something as fundamental as my sobriety would set me up for failure, because I would also accept mediocrity in other areas of my life, including my career. That divine syllogism of drinking = cheating = mediocrity = failure really captured my attention.

I scheduled a private visitation with a priest, who served as the director of Manresa. I wanted to get his opinion on whether or not God had actually spoken to me. The first thing I noticed when I sat down in his office was a group of books on his bookshelf that dealt with alcoholism. They were the same titles on alcoholism that I was familiar with. In our conversation, I found out that he had recently stopped drinking himself. This was no coincidence. God had talked to me. I couldn't address the other issues in my life until I addressed my own substance use. This priest recently passed away, but the enormous benefits of his ministry to the retreatants at Manresa and the poor in New Orleans, endure.

Your midlife tune-up will not be complete until you develop a regular spiritual practice. Whether it is through an organized religion or an individual type of spiritual discipline, the benefits are multifold. This calming of the mind, this getting in touch with and turning things over to your Higher Power, often stops the insanity in life and leads you to truly realize your dreams.

Your Spiritual Purpose Is to Get in Touch with Your Higher Power

> I could prove God statistically.
>
> —George Gallup

There are numerous terms for tapping into your Higher Power. Contemplative prayer is but one of them, as you meditate and contemplate your point in life. Another is discernment, as you pray for decision making. Your Higher Power can help you separate the wheat from the chaff, really deciding in your life what is important and what needs to be discarded. How often do we spend time on things that are not really that important? We worry ourselves with trivialities while we ignore the big picture. One cannot lead an adequate life without a spiritual dimension. This spiritual dimension causes us to appreciate our Higher Power and to connect with life on a higher plane.

The truly spiritual people you meet are usually very happy. This is because they understand the big picture as well as the sacredness of the individual moment. They understand that life is the connection of such moments and that each one is important. They understand that there is a higher plane of existence and that much of what occurs in the earthly world is inconsequential. The spiritually enriched take life a day at a time, experience the moment, have the patience to see the big picture, enjoy everyday activities that others find boring, look for the good in everyone, don't have to be lauded, and are sincere in their lives. Those who are truly spiritually grounded have the perspective, commitment, and calling to succeed in daily life. They are not battered by the slings and arrows of outrageous fortune but confidently and successfully live their lives.

By remaining in touch with your Higher Power, you can find not only tremendous peace but also a system to guide your decisions in everyday life. The key is to make your spiritual practice work for you.

An excellent way to evaluate your purpose is by analyzing it in light of *The Spiritual Exercises* of St. Ignatius of Loyola.

1. God created us that we might know, love, and serve him in this life and be happy with him forever. *This is our goal.*

2. God's purpose in creating us is to draw forth from us a responsive love and service here on earth, so *that we may attain our goal of everlasting happiness with him* in heaven.

3. All the things in this world are gifts of God, created for us, to be *the means* by which we can come to know him better, love him more surely, and serve him more faithfully.

4. As a result, we ought to appreciate and *use these gifts of God*

insofar as they help us towards our goal of loving service and union with God.

5. But insofar as any created things *hinder our progress* towards our goal, we ought to let them go.

6. In everyday life, then, we should *keep ourselves indifferent or undecided* in the face of all created gifts when we have an option and we do not have the clarity of what would be a better choice.

7. We *ought not be led by our natural likes and dislikes* even in matters such as health or sickness, wealth or poverty, between living in the East or in the West, becoming an accountant or lawyer.

8. Rather *our only desire and our one choice should be* an option that better leads us to *the goal* to which God created us.

Empower Yourself with a Regular Spiritual Practice

Therefore, whoever hears the sayings of mine, and does them, I will liken him to a wise man who built his house on the rock: and the rain descended, the floods came, and the winds blew and beat on that house; and it did not fall, for it was founded on the rock.

—Matt. 7:24-25

These things I have spoken unto you, that in me ye might have peace. In the world ye shall have tribulation: but be of good cheer; I have overcome the world.

—John 16:33

As the quote from John points out, the world is full of tribulation, but through God and Jesus, it is possible to overcome your worldly problems and have peace in your life. You can greatly empower yourself with a regular spiritual practice. Too often, we turn to God as a last resort instead of as a first resort. However, by building your life on a foundation of faith, you can equip yourself to handle life's many challenges. The truth is that God wants you to be successful in your life. He wants you to have a good life, good marriage, and good career as well as be active and respected in your community.

However, God won't do this for you. You have to empower

yourself spiritually and construct your own spiritual foundation. "But be doers of the word, and not hearers only, deceiving yourselves" (James 1:22). And this strong spiritual foundation can help ensure that you'll withstand the storms of life.

The proper foundation is built by studying the Bible and being receptive to the Word of God. "In the beginning was the Word, and the Word was with God, and the Word was God. He was in the beginning with God" (John 1:1-2). God's word is alive and powerful, "sharper than any two-edged sword, piercing even to the division of the soul and spirit, . . . and is a discerner of the thoughts and intents of the heart." Finally, the Word of God serves as a guide to us: "Your word is a lamp to my feet and a light to my path."

A proper spiritual foundation not only empowers us against misfortune but also against temptation and evil in the world. Every day we are faced with temptations as well as detours and distractions from our purpose and priorities. Often, these temptations can appear quite innocuous.

While at Manresa one year, I was instructed by an exceptional retreat master who spoke about the origins of evil in society. Many feel that evil began with Lucifer, the former archangel who was cast out of heaven by God and who today is synonymous with Satan. The term Lucifer stands for "light bearer" or "someone who holds the light." Often we can be led astray by the light or tricked by something that looks good on the surface. In this regard, the devil is our "enemy," much like a military commander looking for our weakness. Because we are human, we have a spiritual Achilles' heel that could cause us to stumble on our spiritual path. We are very susceptible to the enemy. The enemy's negative influence on our life could be as harmless as steering us to the second-best choice in a particular situation. You might ask yourself, what's so bad about second best? But it can end up leading you far astray, as it did a prominent member of this retreat master's congregation. The gentleman was happily married with a wonderful family, successful in business, and well respected in the community and church. How could such an upstanding citizen be caught up in an affair with his much younger secretary? The executive lamented that their illicit union started so innocently. The young woman had just broken up with her boyfriend and was very upset. He noticed her dismay and called her into his office to offer consolation. One day, she had a headache and he offered her an aspirin. He sometimes gave her a friendly hug to show support. Then one day, she came into his office and claimed she was not feeling well. Rather than call her a cab, he kindly offered to drive her home. And what began as a show of sympathy eventually led to adultery through a series of bad choices, none of which individually was wrong but none of which was the best course of action. This demonstrates how easily we can be tempted and misled.

The retreat master also related a very moving story about 9/11, the epitome of evil in our lifetime. He mentioned that he happened to be in New York several weeks after the horrific event and wanted to pray for the victims. However, physically reaching ground zero involved no fewer than seven barriers of security. But somehow, thanks to his sincere demeanor, clerical collar, and sheer determination, he was able to pass through all of them and offer a prayer at the site of the tragedy. Each security point was manned by NYPD officers, private security, or the FBI. Each one was a test that required some explanation and persuasion on his part. But God was helping him along the way. At each checkpoint there was suspicion and questions but ultimately the decision to let him continue. One police officer softened up and asked the priest to pray for his nephew, who was lost in the tragedy. The boy had grown up in a tough New Jersey neighborhood, the son of parents with modest means. However, he persevered and worked his way through school, eventually ending up on Wall Street. His family and neighbors were so proud of him and had supported him. At the next security barrier, the guard initially refused him but then relented when coaxed by a co-worker.

The final checkpoint was manned by the excavation crew. When the clergyman walked up, he was approached brusquely by the burly foreman, who appeared both fatigued by his grim task as well as angry at the interruption. How did the priest manage to get past all of the security in the first place? He told the priest that there was too much debris to possibly walk out to the site. At first, the priest couldn't believe that he had come so far only to be turned away. However, to his surprise, the foreman motioned for a bulldozer to come over and transport him out to the center.

Even the driver of the bulldozer had a story of how 9/11 affected him and his neighbors. When he reached the middle of the site, the priest opened his Bible, steadied himself on the front of the bulldozer, and began to pray. All of the excavation work came to a halt and the other workmen joined him in solemn prayer. The priest had empowered himself to fulfill his spiritual purpose at ground zero.

Plan Your Regular Spiritual Practice

> The supreme reality of our time is our indivisibility as children of God and the common vulnerability of our planet.
> —John F. Kennedy

A regular spiritual practice includes spending some time each day in quiet reflection to provide yourself spiritual nourishment as well as ground yourself spiritually. Reflect on your spiritual life on a daily basis. Although you might attend church services weekly, it still helps to enter into a daily dialogue with your Higher Power. One model for a daily spiritual practice is inspired by St. Ignatius of Loyola.

- Take time to thank God for the good things that came into the day. Thank God for the sunshine and the rain, the happy phone call, feeling good all day long, and the energy to perform your job.
- After thanking God, ask for discernment to see clearly and hope that you are growing more fully alive in God and his gifts.
- Examine carefully what acts, omissions, thoughts, and desires tell you about your relationship with God and with yourself and others in God. Think of the times you may have lost your temper, spent too much time on a simple task, or resisted making a decision. Patiently ask yourself what the pattern means about your belief in God and trust in God's love.
- Take what you learned to prayer and speak to God. Speak to God in your own language. Let God surprise you with insight and console you with faith and hope. Bring to God your larger needs, such as an old resentment or a cunning or insidious habit that you badly want to rid yourself of or mindless living throughout

the day without thanking and praising the Creator.

- Determine to keep your spirit filled with gratitude, and take steps to rid yourself of the mindsets that stand between you and the Creator. Decide to change your attitude, shake off a fear, and grow in some special way. Offer this larger movement in life to your Creator.

Another way to commit to a spiritual way of life is to really understand forgiveness. Earlier in this book, we discussed forgiveness as very important for your emotional health as well as supportive to your relationships. The three aspects of forgiveness are empathy, love, and forgetting.

With respect to empathy, forgiveness cannot occur until you can identify with the other person and realize that you make mistakes too. When you pray for someone else to receive grace, you also receive insight on how God helps us all grow. Empathy is the first step towards forgiveness.

The next step is love. Love is the single greatest source of forgiveness and love is blind. Peter came to Jesus and asked, "Lord, how many times should I forgive my brother when he sins against me? Up to seven times?" Jesus responded, "I tell you not seven times but seventy times seven times."

The final aspect of forgiveness is forgetting or letting go, which can often be the most demanding step. This does not necessarily involve suppressing your feelings but allowing any residual negative feelings to leave your heart.

A plan for a regular spiritual practice also involves embracing a God-filled life. God creates every moment and God creates a world that generally is good. Love and find God in all of your relationships. Be aware every moment of every day that there is a voice working on us, pulling us to either the spiritual consolations of God's presence in our lives or a spiritual desolation where we feel distance from God or abandoned.

Spiritual commitment confirms a basic choice we have been making for a long time. Am I going to reach for power or am I going to open myself to love? Will I fight for control over my life or yield to the demands of love?

Those who reach for power want, more than anything else, control over their lives and refuse to let others' needs influence their decisions. They may drag their families all around the country for the sake of job promotions or simply refuse to spend enough time with their children because they work twelve to fourteen hours a day. They want complete control of their time. They also keep tight control over their opinions, refusing to let friends' convictions truly influence them or staying far away from the church's teaching.

Those who choose control tend to tell very little about themselves. They keep their own counsel and are rarely open and frank with others, including their spouses. They feel that self-revelation threatens their control over themselves and others. They ordinarily have a difficult time with authority, perhaps criticizing and ignoring their superiors or manipulating them through passive-aggressive behavior. Above all, they try to keep an upper hand in their friendships. They do not allow themselves to be vulnerable to others. They may help others when they are in need, but they want to choose the time and place for their assistance. Those who opt for power isolate themselves but do not really confront their brokenness.

However, those who choose the way of love know their own brokenness, and out of that humbling knowledge they let the spirit of life lead them to grow. They are open to friendship and also intimacy. Those who choose the way of love are very active in forming and enjoying friendships. They come to know at a deep level that they need to avoid the selfishness that ruins friendships. They risk being vulnerable, growing and changing under the influence of their friends and colleagues. At some point, if they are married, they recognize they have to give up possessing the other and allow their spouse to be themselves. As they grow in the love of God, they see that some friendships focus on doing and making, but others relate almost exclusively to humanness. They continually deepen their compassion.

They experience powerlessness again and again, always finding it difficult and always finding truth in the experience. They are glad just to live and work with those whom God puts into their lives. When asked to take on some authority, they are generally convinced they can help people and are concerned about serving and getting the job done.

Planning for a regular spiritual practice can bring much order into your life and allow you to take things in stride. Often life's struggles are caused by our own blinders, as we see things only from our own point of view. Frequently, it is only through divine guidance that we are able to see certain errors in our perception and understand the entire universe. Only God has the true omniscient point of view, seeing what is down the road and what is truly in our best interest. God has put us all on this earth to achieve a particular purpose. Yet we need to remain spiritually attuned to his will in order to do so. We may have our own ideas of success but need to yield to our Creator. Rather than lament giving up control, we can feel great relief as well as empowered by putting our problems in God's hands. How often have you worried about things that worked out in the end? "Let go and let God" is a credo that can help us so much if we incorporate it in our lives. It's a spiritual power available to us all if we will use it.

Even as I compose this passage, which happens to be on a Sunday, I have to be mindful of this spiritual release in my own life. Lately I had been particularly bothered by a work problem and allowed it to affect my life. Karen and I had attended services earlier today and she could tell that something was bothering me during the mass. "What's wrong?" she whispered. "Just thinking about work," I replied. We happened to be sitting in the first row of the church. Karen pointed at the large cross with Jesus at the front of the altar. "Leave your problems with Jesus," she instructed. I did and was able to enjoy a Sunday for the first time in a long time.

A plan for a regular spiritual practice can involve prayer, meditation, or some other type of contemplation exercise. Your plan can include anything that allows you to pause and reflect. Slowing down to reflect and seek spiritual renewal can be difficult for the busy person. But it is well worth the effort.

A Regular Spiritual Practice Provides Perspective

> Don't let me get me.
> I'm my own worst enemy.
> Don't wanna be my friend no more.
> I wanna be somebody else.
>
> —Pink

We all go through particularly difficult periods in our lives, and I am no exception. My times of greatest anguish were when I felt I was "going against the grain." A regular spiritual practice provided me with the perspective that God had a plan for me. Rather than force God's plan into my life, I had to listen to the clues and feel what He wanted for me. I often became impatient and upset when things didn't work out as I wanted. I particularly experienced a painful state of disconnect when I felt that my career was going awry. I would often question God and wonder where He was when I really needed Him. Finally, as I began to trust in God's wisdom and goodness, I realized that many of his decisions were made in my best interest and that God was looking out for me much more than I'd ever realized. This perspective provided a much more peaceful view of life, that God was, in fact, looking out for me and things would work out for the best.

Spiritual perspective involves understanding that things happen for a reason and work out the way they are generally supposed to. Too often we spend our time railing about what happened rather than trying to find the lesson offered. We spend far too much time comparing ourselves to others, wondering why we are not enjoying the same good fortune. Instead, we should be thankful for the gifts and opportunities we have. We all have more blessings than we are sometimes willing to acknowledge. Despite any past setbacks, if you have your health, you are living and working in the most affluent society in the world. Sure, it would be nice to have more, but be thankful for what you have. Like everyone, I have often taken things for granted, ranging from my health to the love and support of my family to the good people in my life. Taking the time to enjoy and be thankful for your blessings provides spiritual perspective.

In addition, once I believed that my life is to a large extent in God's hands and things would work out, it made me more willing to take risks. These were not foolish risks but those that were consistent with my purpose. When I felt that I was proceeding in accordance with God's plan, I experienced tremendous serenity in my life. A regular spiritual practice helped to provide me with the perspective to understand that I was just a small part of the universe and my actions were in the context of a greater purpose. Discernment or asking for guidance is a very important part of contemplative prayer, as it allows our spiritual power to lead us in the direction of our heart's desire.

Spiritual Perseverance

> He who desires to see the living God face to face should not seek Him in the empty firmament of his mind, but in human love.
>
> —Fyodor Dostoevsky

> We also rejoice in our sufferings because we all know that suffering produces perseverance; perseverance, character, and character, hope. And hope does not disappoint us, because God has poured out his love into our hearts by the Holy Spirit, whom he has given us.
>
> —Rom. 5:3-5

Spiritual perseverance consists of both patience and faith. We have to be patient that God's delays are not necessarily God's denials. Faith sustains us during difficult times with the belief that things will work out for the best and are proceeding according to a divine plan. During my most difficult times, my faith helped me persevere. I would pray for guidance and never was denied. More than anything else, my spiritual perseverance kept me from throwing in the towel. I trusted in God's will and had faith that my Higher Power was looking out for me. Often it is difficult to persevere with prayer, but after the darkness comes the dawn. Persevere.

Midlife Tune-Up Guide

Don't be "consistent," but be simply true.

—Oliver Wendell Holmes

Keeping It All Together

One of the most difficult things in any self-improvement program is to maintain consistency. I have gone through programs where I had an elaborate color scheme for highlighting all of my goals, and I have gone through others that were very simple. I found that a simple program works best. I discussed much of this in the planning chapter, which involved prioritizing your long-term objectives, breaking them into to specific goals and activities, and scheduling the activities. It is really not that difficult, but it is hard to stay on track. You are going to be tempted to backslide. In fact, the temptation will be overwhelming. Don't be surprised if you lose ground here and there. That is natural.

One of the secrets to successful goal setting is setting goals that are just out of reach but not out of sight. I found that when I had too many things on my plate, and set goals too high in the sky, I had the most trouble making progress. The goals were unrealistic and I was not focused. Another secret is learning to reward yourself when you do something right. This positively reinforces good behavior. Also, it is useful to examine your long-term goals periodically, perhaps monthly or quarterly, and see where you are. Then make more plans. Finally, it's sometimes best to have a not-to-do list as opposed to a to-do list. Remain focused and in a good place by ridding your life of time-consuming activities that hold little or no value for you. These can often sap your energy and will as well as decimate your time.

I have provided this appendix to summarize some of the lessons of this book as well as help provide the outline for

your personal tune-up plan. Take some time to read through
the appendix and prepare your own plan.

> Hit the ball over the fence and you can take your time
> going around the bases.
>
> —John W. Raper

Emotional Tune-Up

Passion	1. Develop a passion for living. 2. Remove obstacles from your passion.
Purpose	1. Strive for happiness, well-being. 2. Reduce stress. 3. Overcome negative feelings, doubt, and insecurity.
Power	1. Focus on internal control mechanisms. 2. Understand "emotional intelligence."
Planning	1. Spend time alone, attend a retreat sponsored by a church organization. 2. If you have an issue, check out a support group. 3. Schedule relaxation activities such as massages. 4. Read books from Appendix B.
Perspective	1. Be empathetic. 2. Keep emotional upsets in perspective.
Perseverance	1. Recognize that emotional wholeness and well being is a life long process.

Financial Tune-Up

Passion	1. Change from scarcity consciousness to abundance.
Purpose	1. Seek financial independence. 2. Seek an enjoyable lifestyle at retirement.
Power	1. Become financially literate. 2. Research investment advisors. 3. Watch financial programs. 4. Develop confidence in your financial ability.
Planning	1. Meet with a financial advisor to establish a savings and investment plan. 2. Prepare a budget (remember to pay yourself first).
Perspective	1. Save and invest for the long term.
Perseverance	1. Stick to your budget. 2. Continue to invest even during difficult times.

Career Tune-Up

Passion	1. Find a job that you love. **OR** 2. Find passion in your current job.
Purpose	1. Open your own business. **OR** 2. Recharge your career, redefine your focus.
Power	1. Overcome fear of self-employment. 2. Empower yourself with knowledge. 3. Seek additional responsibilities or opportunities in your current line of work.

Planning	1. Write a business plan. 2. Research a business **OR** 3. Determine how you can provide the most value to your company. 4. Commit one hour per day to improving yourself. 5. Read periodicals in your field.
Perspective	1. Understand that a properly planned business has at least an even chance of success. **OR** 2. View the larger plan for your occupation and where you fit in in terms of value creation.
Perseverance	1. Recognize that it takes three to five years for a new business to be successful. **OR** 2. Resolve to continually improve yourself in your career.

Relationship Tune-Up

Passion	1. Keep the romance in your relationship.
Purpose	1. Improve the quality of your relationship. **OR** 2. Develop a new relationship.
Power	1. Commit to improving your relationship (including acknowledging your own faults). 2. Give of yourself.
Planning	1. Schedule date nights. 2. Resolve to communicate better with your spouse. 3. Do something nice for your spouse every day.
Perspective	1. Empathize with others' points of view.
Perseverance	1. Dedicate yourself to improving or starting a relationship.

Physical Tune-Up

Passion	1. Create physical vigor and passion.
Purpose	1. Adopt a healthy lifestyle. 2. Commit to a regular exercise and diet program.
Power	1. Empower and energize yourself with proper diet and exercise.
Planning	1. Join a gym. 2. Drink a meal replacement for one meal, eat salad for lunch, and replace fats with complex carbohydrates. 3. Shop at the perimeter of the grocery store.
Perspective	1. Set realistic expectations. 2. Don't compare your physique to others. 3. View exercise and a proper diet as permanent lifestyle changes.
Perseverance	1. Avoid perennial New Year's resolutions. 2. Persevere with your lifestyle changes.

Mental Tune-Up

Passion	1. Keep your mind stimulated with a passion for learning.
Purpose	1. Commit to lifelong learning. 2. Leverage down time and driving to help you achieve your purpose.
Power	1. Knowledge = power in the Information Age.
Planning	1. Follow the five-step learning plan.
Perspective	1. Be selective with your learning. 2. Establish user-friendly methods of knowledge retrieval.
Perseverance	1. Persevere in your lifelong quest for knowledge.

Spiritual Tune-Up

Passion	1. Develop a spiritual passion for God in your life.
Purpose	1. Live a God-centered life.
Power	1. Tap into the spiritual power of God by committing to a regular spiritual practice. 2. Empower yourself with forgiveness and love. 3. Live a spiritually attuned life.
Planning	1. Meditate daily. 2. Attend services weekly.
Perspective	1. Understand God's plan in your life. 2. Be thankful for God's many blessings in your life.
Perseverance	1. Realize that God's delays are not God's denials, persevere.

Reading List

Below is a recommended reading list to assist with your tune-up process.

General

Canfield, Jack, and Mark Victor Hanson. *Chicken Soup for the Soul: Living Your Dreams*. 10th anniversary ed. Deerfield Beach, Fla.: Health Communications, 2003.

Chopra, Deepak. *Ageless Body, Timeless Mind*. New York: Harmony, 1993.

Drucker, Peter. *The Effective Executive*. New York: Harper & Row, 1967.

Dychtwald, Ken. *Age Wave: How the Most Important Trend of Our Time Can Change Your Future*. New York: Bantam, 1990.

Frankl, Victor. *Man's Search for Meaning*. Boston: Beacon, 1992.

Peale, Norman Vincent. *The Power of Positive Thinking*. New York: Fawcett Columbine, 1952.

Robbins, Anthony. *Awaken the Giant Within: How to Take Control of Your Mental, Emotional, Physical and Financial Destiny!* New York: Summit, 1991.

Emotional Tune-Up

Bassett, Lucinda. *From Panic to Power: Proven Techniques to Calm Your Anxieties, Conquer Your Fears, and Put You in Control of Your Life*. New York: HarperCollins, 1997.

Dyer, Wayne W. *Your Erroneous Zones*. New York: Funk & Wagnalls, 1976.

Goleman, Daniel. *Emotional Intelligence*. New York: Bantam, 1995.

Hay, Louise. *You Can Heal Your Life*. Santa Monica: Hay, 1998.

Jeffers, Susan J. *Feel the Fear and Do It Anyway*. San Diego: Harcourt Brace Jovanovich, 1987.

Financial Tune-Up

Edelman, Ric. *Ordinary People, Extraordrinary Wealth.* New York: HarperCollins, 2001.

Hill, Napoleon. *Think and Grow Rich.* Hollywood: Wilshire, 1966.

Kiyosaki, Robert T. *Rich Dad, Poor Dad.* 1998. Reprint, New York: Warner, 2000.

Le Boeuf, Michael. *The Millionaire In You: Ten Things You Need to Do Now to Have Maoney and Time to Enjoy It.* New York: Crown Business, 2002.

Stanley, Thomas J. *The Millionaire Mind.* Kansas City: Andrews McMeel, 2000.

————. *The Millionaire Next Door.* Atlanta: Longstreet, 1996.

Career Tune-Up

Ziglar, Zig. *See You at the Top.* 25th anniversary ed. Gretna, La.: Pelican, 2000.

Relationship Tune-Up

Boteach, Shmuley. *Why Can't I Fall in Love?* New York: ReganBooks, 2001.

De Angelis, Barbara. *Are You the One for Me?* New York: Delacorte, 1992.

Gray, John. *Men Are from Mars, Women Are from Venus.* New York: HarperCollins, 1992.

Physical Tune-Up

Phillips, Bill. *Body for Life.* New York: HarperCollins, 1999.

Shilstone, Mackie. *Maximum Energy for Life: A 21-Day Strategic Plan to Feel Great, Reverse the Aging Process, and Optimize Your Health.* Hoboken: Wiley, 2003.

Mental Tune-Up

Tracy, Brian. *Maximum Achievement: Strategies and Skills that Will Unlock Your Hidden Powers to Succeed.* New York: Simon & Schuster, 1993.

Spiritual Tune-Up

Holy Bible, any version.

Peck, M. Scott. *The Road Less Traveled and Beyond: Spiritual Growth in an Age of Anxiety.* New York: Simon & Schuster, 1997.

Warren, Rick. *Daily Inspiration for the Purpose Driven Life: Scriptures and Reflections from the 40 Days of Purpose.* Grand Rapids, Mich.: Inspirio, 2003.

Acknowledgments

Let me first thank all of the people at Pelican Publishing Company for their assistance, starting with Dr. Milburn and Nancy Calhoun, the owners; Nina Kooij, editor in chief; and Karen Robicheaux, promotion assistant.

Thanks also to Mary Karl, Amy Parker, and Cheryl Frame, who helped with typing and revisions. Thanks also to Ezra Hodge, Pam Egan, and Louisette Kidd. Thanks also to Michael LeBouef, for his support and guidance. Special thanks to Kristin McLaren, who went over and above the call of duty in helping me with editing and illustrations.

Special appreciation to my wife, Karen, for enduring a political campaign as well as the completion of this book during our courtship.